Cardiac Imaging THE REQUISITES

SERIES EDITOR **James H. Thrall,** MD
Radiologist-in-Chief
Department of Radiology
Massachusetts General Hospital
Juan M. Taveras Professor of Radiology
Harvard Medical School
Boston, Massachusetts

OTHER VOLUMES IN THE REQUISITES™ SERIES

Gastrointestinal Radiology

Pediatric Radiology

Neuroradiology

Nuclear Medicine

Ultrasound

Musculoskeletal Radiology

Genitourinary Radiology

Thoracic Radiology

Breast Imaging

Vascular and Interventional Radiology

Emergency Radiology

Cardiac Imaging

THE REQUISITES

Second Edition

Stephen Wilmot Miller, M.D.
Associate Professor of Radiology
Harvard Medical School
Massachusetts General Hospital
Boston, Massachusetts

with 894 illustrations

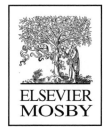

ELSEVIER
MOSBY

ELSEVIER
MOSBY

The Curtis Center
170 S Independence Mall W 300E
Philadelphia, Pennsylvania 19106

THE REQUISITES™
THE REQUISITES
THE REQUISITES
THE REQUISITES
THE REQUISITES

THE REQUISITES is a proprietary trademark
of Mosby, Inc.

Notice

Radiology is an ever-changing field. Standard safety precautions must be followed,
but as new research and clinical experience broaden our knowledge, changes in
treatment and drug therapy may become necessary or appropriate. Readers are
advised to check the most current product information provided by the
manufacturer of each drug to be administered to verify the recommended dose,
the method and duration of administration, and contraindications. It is the
responsibility of the treating physician, relying on experience and knowledge of
the patient, to determine dosages and the best treatment for each individual
patient. Neither the Publisher nor the editor assumes any liability for any injury
and/or damage to persons or property arising from this publication.

The Publisher

Previous edition copyrighted 1998

Acquisitions Editor: Hilarie Surrena

Printed in the United States of America

Last digit is the print number: 9   8   7   6   5   4   3   2   1

To *Richard L. Liberthson M.D.* and *Roman W. DeSanctis M.D.*
Outstanding cardiologists and educators at the Massachusetts General Hospital

S.W.M.

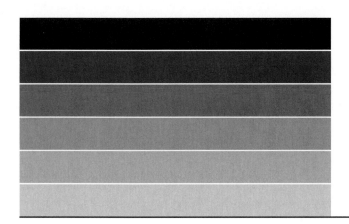

Contributors

Suhny Abbara, M.D.
Cardiac Radiologist
Director of Non Invasive Cardiovascular Imaging
Department of Radiology
Massachusetts General Hospital
Boston, Massachusetts

Lawrence M. Boxt, M.D.
Chief, Division of Cardiovascular Imaging
Beth Israel Medical Center
Professor of Clinical Radiology
Albert Einstein College of Medicine
Yeshiva University
New York, New York

Mary Etta E. King, M.D.
Associate Professor of Pediatrics
Harvard Medical School
Director, Pediatric Echocardiography
Massachusetts General Hospital
Boston, Massachusetts

Stephen Wilmot Miller, M.D.
Associate Professor of Radiology
Harvard Medical School
Massachusetts General Hospital
Boston, Massachusetts

Stefan Mark Nidorf, M.D., M.B.B.S., F.R.A.C.P., F.A.C.C.
Cardiologist
Department of Cardiovascular Medicine
Sir Charles Gardiner Hospital
Queen Elizabeth II Medical Centre
Perth, Western Australia

John G. Santilli, M.D.
Assistant Professor of Radiology
Harvard Medical School
Department of Radiology
Massachusetts General Hospital
Children's Hospital Boston
Boston, Massachusetts

Stephan Wicky, M.D.
Associate Professor
Harvard Medical School
Director Clinical Cardiovascular Radiology
Department of Radiology
Massachusetts General Hospital
Boston, Massachusetts

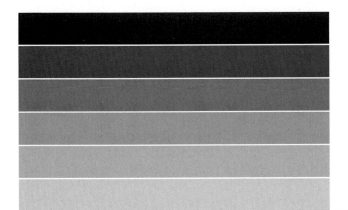

Foreword

The second edition of *Cardiac Imaging: THE REQUISITES* continues the theme of THE REQUISITES series. It is a practical, concise yet remarkably comprehensive text equally useful for residents and fellows during their training and by physicians involved in cardiac imaging seeking to review or expand their knowledge.

Cardiac imaging is an enormously important topic in medicine because of the prevalence of cardiovascular disease including coronary artery disease in society. It is also a very challenging topic from the perspective of the multiple methods that are required for a comprehensive approach to imaging of the heart and its associated vessels. Therefore, the task of developing a concise book is challenging. Dr. Steven Wilmot Miller has again done an outstanding job in ably rising to this challenge along with selected colleagues invited to contribute to this new edition.

Dr. Miller has again structured his book to provide basic information that residents or fellows should master during their training in order to correctly interpret cardiac imaging studies. He and his co-authors expand upon these fundamental principles by addressing questions in clinical context. This of course is very important in heart and coronary artery disease due to the interplay between patient risk factors and findings on imaging evaluations, which must both be taken into account to assess significance.

With respect to the challenge covering the rapidly evolving technology for cardiac imaging, Dr. Miller has systematically included the appropriate new material. The second edition of *Cardiac Imaging: THE REQUISITES* presents critical and exciting new applications using multidetector computed tomography and MRI and MRA of the heart and the aorta. These methods are making a dramatic impact on the way patients are diagnosed and managed. New non invasive approaches are shifting the balance away from the cardiac catheterization laboratory as the location for definitive imaging although conventional coronary angiography remains the gold standard at the present time. Perhaps by the publication of the third edition of *Cardiac Imaging: THE REQUISITES* this will have changed!

The pervasiveness of digital imaging is illustrated in this book by the inclusion of digital coronary angiograms, which were under development but not in widespread use at the time of the first edition. It is now fair to say that cardiac imaging is substantially an all-digital area of practice with the adoption of digital coronary angiography.

THE REQUISITES have now become old friends to a generation of physicians in training and in practice. The original intent of this series was to provide the resident or a fellow with a text that might be reasonably read within several days at the beginning of each rotation and then used for reference and review during subsequent rotations or board preparation. The books in THE REQUISITES series are not intended to be exhaustive but to provide basic conceptual, factual and interpretive material required for clinical practice. Each book is written by a nationally recognized authority and each author is challenged to present material in the context of today's practice of medicine rather than grafting information about new imaging approaches onto older out-of date material.

Dr. Miller and his invited co-authors have done an outstanding job in sustaining the philosophy of THE REQUISITES series and he has produced another truly contemporary text for the cardiac imaging community. I believe that *Cardiac Imaging: THE REQUISITES* will serve residents and fellows as a concise and useful introduction to the subject and will also serve as a very manageable text for reference and review by practicing physicians.

James H. Thrall, M.D.

Radiologist-in-Chief
Massachusetts General Hospital
Juan M. Taveras Professor of Radiology
Harvard Medical School
Boston, Massachusetts

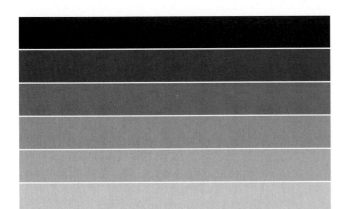

Preface

Cardiovascular disease is the dominant medical disease in most of the developed countries and accounts for almost half of all deaths. In the United States, about 6 million people have some type of cardiovascular disease although the prevalence is decreasing, perhaps because of epidemiological measures to reduce risk factors and after the introduction of new therapies. The keystone of cardiac diagnosis remains imaging, both for the initial diagnosis and for the evaluation of subsequent therapy. Multiple imaging modalities can provide exquisite anatomic detail of the cardiac chambers, coronary arteries, pericardium, and arterial and venous systems. Physiologic information of blood flow and cardiac motion is frequently obtained by various imaging techniques. It is therefore fitting that *The Requisites*, intended to provide core material in major organ systems, include a book on cardiac imaging that can be used by physicians in radiology, cardiology, cardiovascular surgery, pediatrics, and associated subspecialties.

The second edition has been extensively revised with about 300 new illustrations and now covers cardiovascular disease from birth through old age. This edition is upgraded to reflect the current state of the art for medical imaging. The scope has been broadened to include more CT and MRI of the heart and aorta. New topics include MDCT of aortic disease, MRI tensor imaging of pericardial disease, and MRA of valvular heart disease. The chapters on cardiac angiography have been expanded with new illustrations of the digital images obtained in the catheterization laboratory.

Based on the multiple imaging technologies, this volume first presents the essentials of cardiac imaging concepts by modality. Pertinent anatomic and physiologic images are illustrated by chest radiography, echocardiography, magnetic resonance imaging, and angiography. Then based on a "spiral learning" approach, the latter chapters cover subjects by disease, adding more complex concepts.

The format has also been expanded with lists of associated conditions and differential diagnoses. Break-out Boxes have been added for quick reference. I have also constructed short lists of imaging signs and split them into groups by anatomic location, physiology, or pathology for easier recall. For the difficult topic of congenital heart disease, I have developed "Aunt Marys" (Dr. Benjamin Felson's aunt was Minnie; mine is Mary) for images that should be instantly recognized. The name reflects the fact that I do not need to analyze the features of my Aunt Mary minutely to know who she is, in the same way that one should instantly recognize the snowman configuration of total anomalous pulmonary venous connection. Finally, because I believe that learning results when a teacher speaks directly to the students, the style of the book departs from standard medical writing in I frequently use the second person.

Stephen Wilmot Miller, M.D.

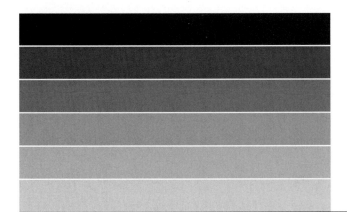

Preface to First Edition

The Requisites in Radiology series was conceived by Dr. James H. Thrall as a set of books that radiology residents would find useful from the first day of their residency through 4 years of training. Based on a "spiral learning" approach, this volume seeks to present core material on the subspecialty and then enhance the information base with more complex concepts. Dr. Thrall asked me to organize a curriculum on cardiovascular imaging, defining the basic knowledge that one should have at the end of a postgraduate radiology residency. *Cardiac Radiology: The Requisites* presents this core knowledge.

The resident in radiology first needs an overview of cardiac radiology with anatomic and physiologic correlations. In that context, the first four chapters of the text feature the essentials of imaging technology for chest film, magnetic resonance imaging, echocardiography, and angiography. Subsequent chapters, organized by common cardiac diseases, build upon these essentials and correlate diagnostic possibilities with clinical context.

The radiology resident also needs to be oriented to the logic of differential diagnosis based on the analysis of the image. The process of making a diagnosis from an image is typically accomplished in two steps. First, the abnormality is detected visually and analyzed by its location, borders, calcification, and other characteristics. Because some diseases form an imaging spectrum as a gradation from normal, this first step of recognizing an abnormality may prove difficult. Shunt vascularity, for example, is a continuum ranging from normal size pulmonary arteries when the shunt is small, to large pulmonary arteries when the pulmonary flow is greater than twice the systemic flow. Further, normal structures must be distinguished from abnormal structures before a diagnosis can have any relevance, although some abnormalities are so unique—the scimitar syndrome—that they have no differential. Second, by deductive reasoning a list matching possible diseases is constructed and then re-ordered to begin with the most likely possibility.

In this text, lists of associated conditions and differential diagnoses are highlighted in breakouts for quick reference. I have also constructed short lists of radiologic signs and split them into groups by location, physiology, or pathology for easier recall. For the difficult topic of congenital heart disease, I have developed "Aunt Mary" (Dr. Benjamin Felson's aunt was Minnie; mine is Mary) for images that should be instantly recognized. The name reflects the fact that I do not need to analyze the features of my Aunt Mary minutely to know who she is, in the same way one should instantly recognize the snowman configuration of total anomalous pulmonary venous connection.

In organizing the content of the book, I have discussed all of the common imaging modalities. I have illustrated most common cardiac diseases, as well, and have included uncommon diseases if the imaging examination is a key to the diagnosis or is so unique that it should be identified as an "Aunt Mary." Clinical and pathologic content is interwoven and correlated with the imaging so that salient points are discussed in the context of a patient's demand for a diagnosis and treatment. Finally, because I believe that good teaching results when the lecturer, seminar leader, or writer speaks directly to the students, the style of the book departs from standard medical writing in that the second person is frequently addressed.

I hope that the curriculum offered in *Cardiac Radiology: The Requisites* becomes a valuable learning tool for all its readers.

Stephen Wilmot Miller, M.D.

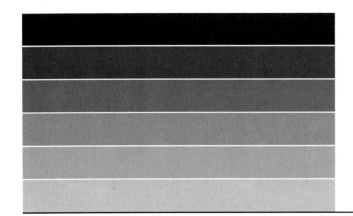

Acknowledgments

Writing a book involves the creative talents of many people who have contributed to the book's organization, content, and illustrations. I would like to thank a number of those involved in the production of the second edition of *Cardiac Imaging: The Requisites*.

Dr. James H. Thrall, Radiologist-in-Chief at the Massachusetts General Hospital and Juan M. Taveras Professor of Radiology at Harvard Medical School, conceived the idea of The Requisites series. I appreciate his support through two editions by providing the academic milieu so that I could write about cardiovascular imaging.

Two colleagues whose friendship covers many years completely rewrote their chapters from the first edition. Dr. Mary Etta E. King's chapter draws on her 30-year experience in echocardiography, having founded the pediatric echocardiography section at the Massachusetts General Hospital. Dr. Lawrence Boxt continues to be one of the innovators in magnetic resonance imaging of the heart.

New authors have added a refreshing collaboration with me in several chapters. Dr. Stephan Wicky, one of the few radiologists who performs cardiac catheterization, has updated the chapters on angiography and ischemic heart disease. Dr. Suhny Abbara has extensive experience in cross-sectional imaging and three-dimensional imaging and has added these modalities to the chapter on pericardial and myocardial imaging. Dr. John Santilli, whose practice includes both pediatric and adult imaging, has added his expertise on imaging the aorta. I thank each for their well-written contributions.

Publishing a book is a team effort of many people at all stages of the production process. First, I want to thank Sara Fogg Crafts for her many contributions ranging from the co-ordination of the initial drafts, working with the editors for standardizing style and format, transcription, and library research. The Philadelphia editors at Elsevier deserve a particular round of applause—Hilarie Surrena for her persistence and belief that the chapters finally would arrive, and Christy Bracken for her meticulous attention to all the details that mark a good publication. Emily McGrath-Christie worked with me as Marketing Manager. Dan Clipner oversaw the production. We authors truly were translated into English! Working in Essex in the United Kingdom, Sukie Hunter and Maureen Allen were our copyeditors.

The photographs in an imaging book are critical to illustrate the text. Kristi Martik and Susanne Loomis at the Radiology Educational Media Services at the Massachusetts General Hospital skillfully converted images from the PACS into Adobe PhotoShop™, clarified details, and printed them electronically. They were also the artists for the new drawings.

Stephen Wilmot Miller, M.D.

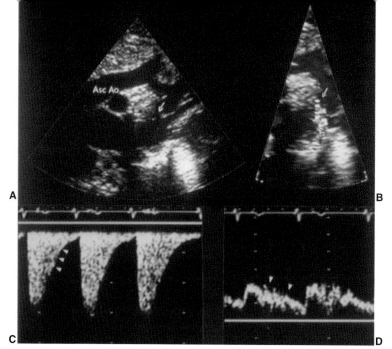

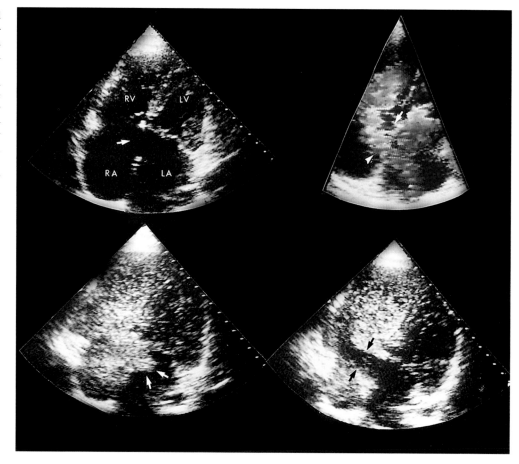

Plate 4 **A,** Suprasternal notch two-dimensional echocardiographic view of the aortic arch demonstrating a discrete narrowing at the aortic isthmus (arrow) indicative of an aortic coarctation. **B,** Color flow Doppler of the same view, which shows flow acceleration and turbulence at the site of the coarctation, where the low velocity blue color seen in the transverse arch turns to a bright blue and yellow jet through the discrete obstruction (arrow). **C,** Continuous wave Doppler tracing in the descending thoracic aorta showing the typical Doppler pattern for coarctation, with high-velocity systolic flow and a slurring of the flow profile (arrows) that reflects continued gradient across the coarctation into diastole. **D,** Pulsed wave Doppler spectral tracing from the abdominal aorta that shows a delay in systolic upstroke, turbulent systolic flow, and continued antegrade flow in diastole, all of which indicate significant flow obstruction in the proximal aorta. Asc Ao, ascending aorta. (With permission from King ME. Echocardiographic evaluation of the adult with unoperated congenital heart disease. In: Otto CM. *Textbook of clinical echocardiography*, 2nd ed. Philadelphia, PA: WB Saunders, 2002.) (This figure is reproduced in black and white on page **77.**)

Plate 5 Series of apical four-chamber echocardiographic views in a patient with an ostium primum atrial septal defect. In the upper left panel, the dropout in the lower atrial septum (arrow) delineates the defect. Doppler color flow mapping (upper right) demonstrates a wide band of flow crossing from the left atrium (LA) to the right atrium (RA; arrows). Following intravenous injection of agitated saline, microbubbles are detected as contrast within the cardiac chambers. In the lower left panel, right-to-left shunting can be seen across the defect (arrows) and left-to-right negative contrast is shown in the lower right panel (arrows) as unopacified blood crosses the atrial defect. LV, left ventricle; RV, right ventricle. (From Levine RA, *et al.* Echocardiography: principles and clinical applications. In: Eagle KA, *et al.*, eds. *The practice of cardiology*. Boston, MA: Little, Brown, 1989.) (This figure is reproduced in black and white on page **78.**)

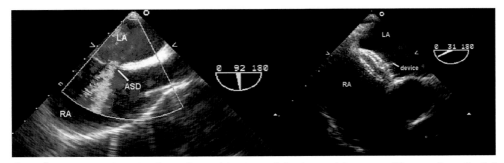

Plate 6 Transesophageal echocardiographic view of the interatrial septum. The panel on the left shows a discrete atrial septal defect (ASD) with color Doppler demonstration of shunting from left (LA) to right atrium (RA). The panel on the right shows a percutaneous closure device occluding the atrial septal defect (arrow). The device is well-aligned along the atrial septum with visualization of both the right and left atrial components. (This figure is reproduced in black and white on page **79**.)

Plate 7 Diagrammatic representation of multiple echocardiographic views of the interventricular septum with color encoding of the subdivisions of the septum. The muscular septum is shown in blue, the inlet septum in green, the infundibular septum in orange, and the membranous septum in red. Ao, aorta; LA, left atrium; LV, left ventricle; PA, pulmonary artery; PV, pulmonary valve; RA, right atrium; RV, right ventricle; RVOT, right ventricular outflow tract. (This figure is reproduced in black and white on page **80**.)

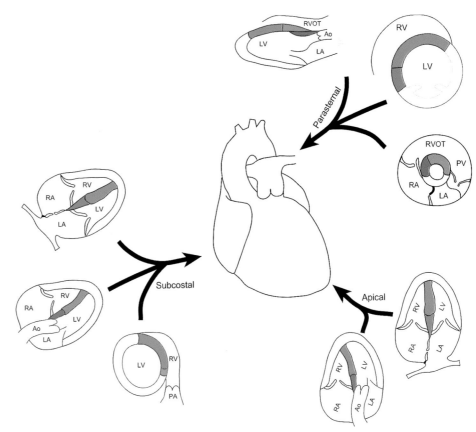

Plate 8 Two-dimensional echocardiographic images and color flow Doppler illustration of shunt flow across small ventricular septal defects (VSDs). **A,** Following repair of a malalignment VSD, a small residual defect is present at the upper edge of the patch (arrow). **B,** The jet of shunt flow is seen as a mosaic-like stream emerging from the right ventricular aspect of the defect. Flow accelerates along the left ventricular septal surface (arrows) as it approaches the defect. **C,** Two small defects in the midmuscular septum are present (arrows). **D,** Two discrete jets can be detected by color Doppler. Ao, aorta; LA, left atrium; LV, left ventricle; RA, right atrium; RV, right ventricle. (This figure is reproduced in black and white on page **82**.)

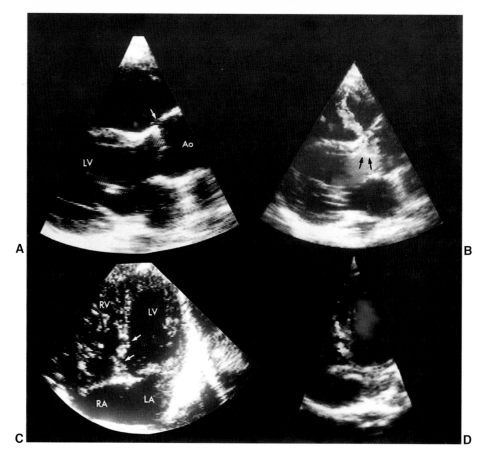

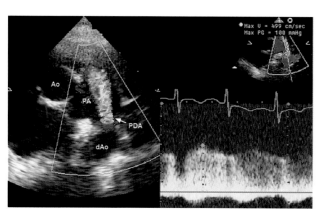

Plate 9 Parasternal short-axis images at the base of the heart depicting flow through a patent ductus arteriosus (PDA) by color Doppler on the left, and the continuous wave Doppler sample of the ductal flow in the panel on the right. The peak velocity of ductal shunt flow is measured at 4.99 m/sec which is equivalent to a 100 mmHg pressure gradient between the aorta (Ao) and pulmonary artery (PA). dAo, descending aorta. (This figure is reproduced in black and white on page **83**.)

Plate 10 **ECG-gated 16-detector row CT coronary angiography.** An isotropic resolution of 0.5 mm is obtained at a temporal resolution of 210 msec, allowing during diastole to image the coronary arteries. Three-dimensional surface rendering reconstruction of the epicardial coronary arteries. (This figure is reproduced in black and white on page **135**.)

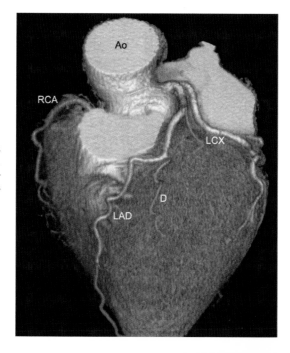

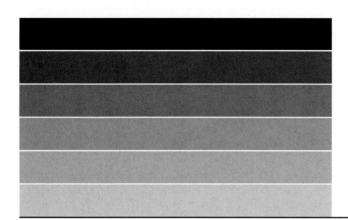

Contents

PART I
IMAGING MODALITIES 1

1 **The Elements of Cardiac Imaging** 3
Stephen Wilmot Miller

2 **Echocardiography** 42
Mary Etta E. King and Stefan Mark Nidorf

3 **Cardiac Magnetic Resonance Imaging** 88
Lawrence M. Boxt

4 **Cardiac Angiography** 132
Stephan Wicky and Stephen Wilmot Miller

PART II
SPECIFIC DISEASES 157

5 **Valvular Heart Disease** 159
Stephen Wilmot Miller

6 **Ischemic Heart Disease** 202
Stephan Wicky and Stephen Wilmot Miller

7 **Pericardial and Myocardial Disease** 245
Suhny Abbara and Stephen Wilmot Miller

8 **Congenital Heart Disease** 284
Stephen Wilmot Miller

9 **Thoracic Aortic Disease** 366
John G. Santilli and Stephen Wilmot Miller

Index 427

IMAGING MODALITIES

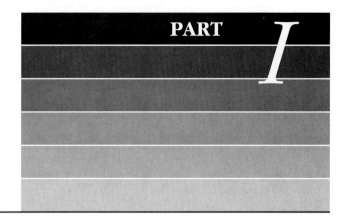

CHAPTER 1

The Elements of Cardiac Imaging

STEPHEN WILMOT MILLER

Cardiac Shape and Size
Age and its Visible Effects
Evaluation of Heart Size
Chamber Enlargement
Cardiac and Pericardial Calcifications
Aortic Valve Calcification
Mitral Annulus Calcification
Mitral Valve Calcification
Myocardial Calcification
Left Atrial Calcification
Pericardial Calcification
Coronary Calcification
Pulmonary Vasculature
Determining the Vascular Pattern
Diminished Vasculature
High-output States
Pulmonary Artery Hypertension
Pulmonary Venous Hypertension
Skeletal Abnormalities in Heart Disease
Cardiac Surgery
Thoracic Cage and Heart Disease
Congenital Syndromes with Heart Disease
The Coronary Sinus and the Left Superior Vena Cava
Coronary Sinus
Left Superior Vena Cava

The anatomic and physiologic effects of heart disease have many common imaging features. Chamber dilatation, valve calcification, and anomalous connections are morphologic signs of cardiac abnormalities. Increased or decreased blood flow and segmental wall motion disorders are physiologic signs of heart disease. The analysis for cardiovascular disease on the chest film, echocardiogram, computed tomography (CT) scan, and magnetic resonance image (MRI) begins with a search for these common elements. Then a more systematic imaging examination can be devised to address particular questions.

The chest film is often the first imaging procedure performed when heart disease is suspected, and, more commonly, it is used to assess and follow the severity of cardiac disease. Because the chest film forms images by projection, this technique detects only those cardiopulmonary abnormalities that change the shape of the heart, mediastinum, and lungs and those that alter the structure of the pulmonary vasculature. Clinically silent heart disease may also be detected on a chest film taken for other reasons. Extracardiac structures, particularly in the abdomen and the thoracic cage, may produce additional clues indicating heart disease. Calcification in the aortic valve, for example, identifies the abnormal structure and directs the differential diagnosis toward a particular pathologic lesion (Box 1-1).

CARDIAC SHAPE AND SIZE

Age and its Visible Effects

The age of the patient greatly influences what is considered the normal appearance of the heart and lungs, and there are some normal variants that may at times mimic disease. In the infant, the thymus typically obscures the upper portion of the mediastinum and may overlay the pulmonary hilum. In rare instances it extends inferiorly,

---

Box 1-1 Analysis of Chest Film for Cardiac Disease

The shape and size of the heart and its individual chambers
The pulmonary vasculature, which mirrors the physiologic pressure and volume state of the cardiopulmonary system
The mediastinum, for the size and location of the aorta and major systemic veins
Extracardiac anomalies that may be associated with heart disease

causing the transverse heart size to appear falsely large. In the first day of life, the pulmonary vasculature has a fuzzy appearance. This normally represents the complex and rapidly changing pressures and flows in the lungs but can suggest pulmonary abnormalities (such as transient tachypnea of the newborn or respiratory distress syndrome) or cardiac disease. In sick children under prolonged stress, the thymus may shrink to a small size but usually is still partially visible. The thymic shadow is invisible in transposition of the great arteries.

In the child and adolescent, the bronchopulmonary markings become more distinguishable, and the thymic shadow regresses and becomes inapparent so you can see the aortic arch and pulmonary trunk. A convex pulmonary trunk in girls in their late teens may suggest pulmonary artery enlargement, but in the absence of a heart murmur this is usually a normal variant (Figure 1-1). However, an ECG may be necessary to exclude entities such as pulmonary stenosis and left-to-right shunts. The "double density" of the pulmonary veins may mimic an enlarged left atrium (Figure 1-2), but a large left atrium has a rounder curve and extends medially above the diaphragm.

In the young adult, the major changes in the cardiac silhouette are the mild prominence of the aortic arch and the vertical orientation of the heart. In the elderly, the thoracic aorta may become elongated and tortuous. The cardiac apex becomes more rounded and the overall heart size is smaller, which possibly reflects aging changes but more probably results from the loss of heart muscle because of lack of exercise.

Evaluation of Heart Size

Cardiothoracic Ratio

The determination of heart size, both subjectively and quantitatively, has been assessed from the chest film for more than 70 years. Then Danzer described the cardiothoracic ratio, which is still one of the most common measurements of overall heart size. This ratio was constructed to measure left ventricular dilation. Because it measures the transverse heart diameter, the cardiothoracic ratio is usually normal when either the left atrium or the right ventricle is moderately enlarged, because neither of these two chambers is reflected in the transverse dimension. The left atrium and right ventricle become border-forming when they are severely enlarged. Rose and colleagues noted that changes in left ventricular volume up to 66% in excess of normal are needed for the cardiothoracic ratio to reliably detect enlargement of the left ventricle (Table 1-1).

When the heart size is subjectively evaluated based on the configuration of the heart with respect to the thorax, the sensitivity and specificity are quite similar to the measured cardiothoracic ratio. For this reason and because quantitative measurements from tomographic imaging methods are commonly available, the cardiothoracic ratio is now used mainly as an adjunct in assessing heart size on the chest film. Although the cardiothoracic ratio is moderately variable among individuals, it is a useful indicator in an individual who is being watched for potential cardiac dilatation, such as in chronic aortic regurgitation. In this instance, an abrupt change in the cardiothoracic ratio suggests the need for urgent clinical reevaluation.

Marathon runners with heart rates in the range of 30–40 beats/min occasionally have a cardiothoracic ratio between 0.50 and 0.55, reflecting the normal physiologic dilatation of the heart rather than any overall hypertrophy.

Several other measurements can be made from the standard posteroanterior and lateral chest film. Examples include total heart volume, left atrial dimension on the frontal film, width of the right descending pulmonary artery, and the distance of the left ventricle behind the inferior vena cava. These, however, are rarely used now in clinical evaluation.

Most measurements made from the chest film have poor correlation with left ventricular size from quantitative angiographic measurements. Therefore, the measurements of specific chamber diameters, volumes, and wall thicknesses should be made from techniques that show

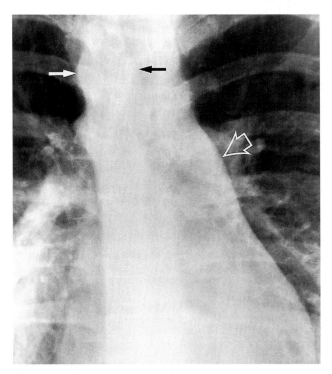

Figure 1-1   Convex main pulmonary artery. The moderate convexity of the main pulmonary artery segment (arrowhead) is a normal variant in this young adult even though the aortic arch (arrows) is on the right side. The space usually occupied by a left aortic arch contains the aberrant left subclavian artery.

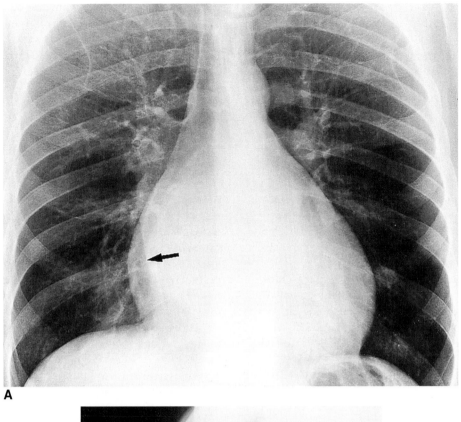

A

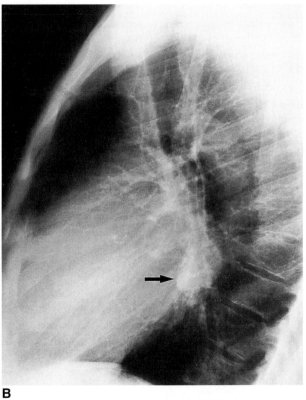

B

Figure 1-2   Confluence of the pulmonary veins. The superior and inferior right pulmonary veins may join and connect with the left atrium as a common vein. This normal variant may look similar to an enlarged left atrium (arrow) on the frontal film (**A**) and a pulmonary nodule (arrow) on the lateral film (**B**).

Table 1-1 Cardiothoracic Ratio

$$\text{Cardiothoracic ratio} = \frac{\text{Widest transverse cardiac diameter}}{\text{Widest inside thoracic diameter}}$$

Patient Characteristics		Normal Ratio
Newborn		< 0.6
>1 month old		< 0.5
Sensitivity	=	0.45 (Many patients with left ventricular dilatation are not detected)
Specificity	=	0.85 (When ratio exceeds the normal value, heart is clearly large)
Accuracy	=	0.59

Modified with permission from Rose CP, Stolberg HO. The limited utility of the plain chest film in the assessment of left ventricular structure and function. *Invest Radiol* 1982;17:139-144.

the chamber cavities (e.g., echocardiography, angiography, and MRI).

Measurements of the heart and mediastinum are dramatically affected by the height of the diaphragm and the intrathoracic pressure and less so by the body position and status of the intravascular volume (Table 1-2).

Chamber Enlargement

Usually the abnormal enlargement of the heart is easily recognized by its displacement out of the mediastinum. It may also be recognized by contour changes, by a new or different interface with the adjacent lung, or by displacement of adjacent mediastinal structures.

Each chamber basically enlarges directly outward from its normal position. Except for the right ventricle, isolated chamber enlargement does not affect the position of the heart in the mediastinum nor the identification of other chamber enlargement. When the right ventricle enlarges, it contacts the sternum and rotates the heart

Box 1-2 Right Ventricular Enlargement on Chest Film

Frontal view
- Rounding of left heart border
- Uplifted apex

Lateral view
- Filling in of retrosternal space
- Rotation of heart posteriorly

posteriorly and in a clockwise direction as viewed from below. Frequently in right ventricular enlargement, the normal left ventricle may falsely appear enlarged on both the frontal and lateral films because the entire heart is displaced posteriorly. If the right ventricle is dilated, the diagnosis of left ventricular enlargement may not be possible in the chest film (Dinsmore's principle). Therefore, you should assess the size of the right ventricle on the lateral film before you judge the left ventricle (Figure 1-3, Box 1-2).

Right Atrium

In the frontal view the right atrium is visible because of its border with the right middle lobe (Box 1-3). Neither subtle nor moderate enlargement can be recognized accurately because there is moderate variability of its shape in normal subjects, and in expiration the right atrium becomes more round and moves to the right (Figures 1-4, 1-5).

The right atrium, as do the other three chambers, enlarges because of increased pressure, increased blood volume, or a wall abnormality. Common causes of right atrial enlargement are tricuspid stenosis and regurgitation, atrial septal defect, atrial fibrillation, and dilated cardiomyopathy. Ebstein's anomaly may have all of these features. In pulmonary atresia, the right atrium dilates in direct proportion to the amount of tricuspid regurgitation (Figure 1-6).

Table 1-2 Typical Variations of Heart and Mediastinum Measurements on the Chest Film

Circumstance	Variation
In expiration	Transverse diameter of heart and mediastinum widens Indistinct appearance of pulmonary hilum can be identical to that seen with pulmonary edema
In recumbent position	Heart is broader Lung volumes are lower Upper lobe arteries and veins appear more distended
On posteroanterior film	Change in heart width between systole and diastole is typically less than 1 cm
On right anterior oblique film	Heart size does not change between systole and diastole Left ventricular apex appears akinetic
On left anterior oblique film	Posterolateral wall motion is typically more than 1 cm

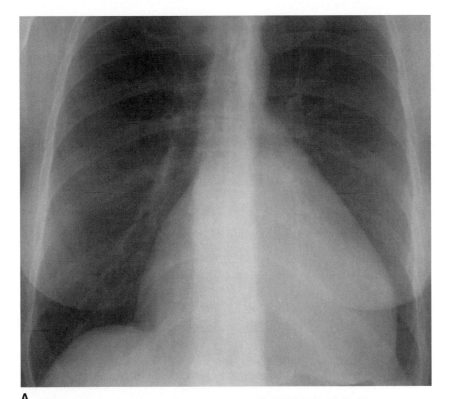

A

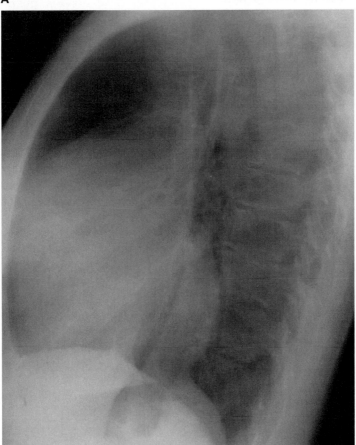

B

Figure 1-3   Right heart enlargement suggesting left heart enlargement. The left ventricle is normal in this patient with Ebstein's anomaly. **A,** The entire left heart border from the pulmonary artery to the diaphragm is the border of the huge right ventricle. **B,** The posterior border of the heart projected over the spine is the normal-sized left ventricle, which has been pushed backward by the anterior right ventricle touching the sternum.

Box 1-3   Right Atrial Enlargement on Chest Film

Displacement of more than several centimeters to the right of the spine (Figure 1-4)

A prominent convexity superiorly near the superior vena caval junction on the frontal film (Figure 1-5)

On the lateral view, a horizontal interface with the lung above the right ventricle (the normal right atrium is not visible in the lateral view)

On the lateral view, displacement of the heart behind the inferior vena cava mimicking left ventricular enlargement

All the signs of right heart enlargement that are implied on the chest film are directly visible on the CT scan. The right atrium and ventricle touch the anterior chest wall and rotate the heart posteriorly. The right coronary artery adjacent to the right atrial appendage lies to the left of the sternum (Figure 1-7).

Right Ventricle

On the lateral view, the normal right ventricle does not touch more than one-quarter of the lower portion of the sternum as measured by the distance from the sternodiaphragmatic angle to the point at which the trachea meets the sternum. One sign of right ventricular enlargement is the filling in of more than one-third of the retrosternal space. On the frontal view, the normal right ventricle is not visible, and only extreme dilatation causes recognizable signs because the heart rotates clockwise as it dilates and pushes against the sternum. In this instance, the usual contour of the left atrial appendage is rotated posteriorly and is no longer part of the left side of the mediastinum. You can recognize this sign by an unusually long convex curvature extending inferiorly from the main pulmonary artery (Figure 1-8). In extreme instances the entire left heart border may be the right ventricle (Box 1-2).

In tetralogy of Fallot when the fat pad is absent in the left cardiophrenic angle, the heart may have an uplifted cardiac apex (Figure 1-9), which has been called the "boot-shaped heart" or the *coeur en sabot*. The right ventricle is not enlarged but may have hypertrophy.

Common causes of right ventricular enlargement are pulmonary valve stenosis, pulmonary artery hypertension (cor pulmonale), atrial septal defect, tricuspid regurgitation, and dilated cardiomyopathy; it can occur secondarily to left ventricular failure.

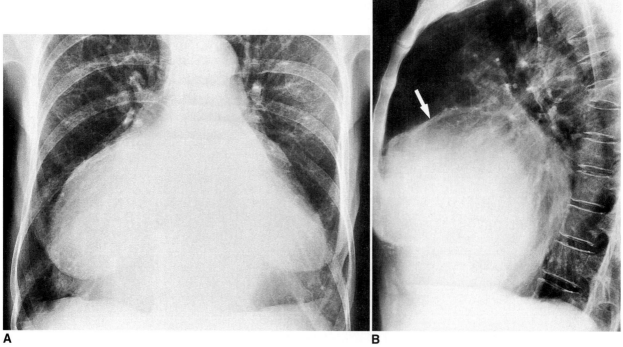

A   **B**

Figure 1-4   Right atrial enlargement in rheumatic heart disease. A, The unusually large right atrium compresses the right middle lobe and extends inferiorly to intersect the diaphragm. A large left atrium usually does not have a diaphragmatic interface. **B,** Enlargement of the right heart creates a sharp interface with the lung (arrow). The horizontal contour suggests that this is the right atrial appendage rather than the right ventricle.

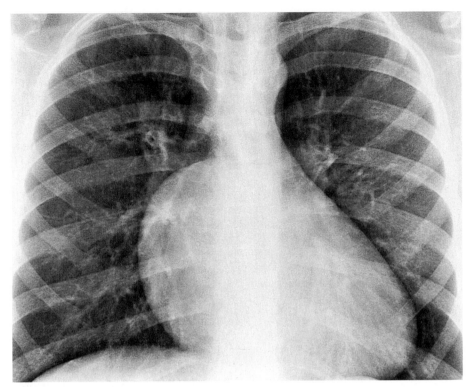

Figure 1-5   Superior right atrial convexity. In Ebstein's anomaly, the large right atrium has a characteristic round superior border.

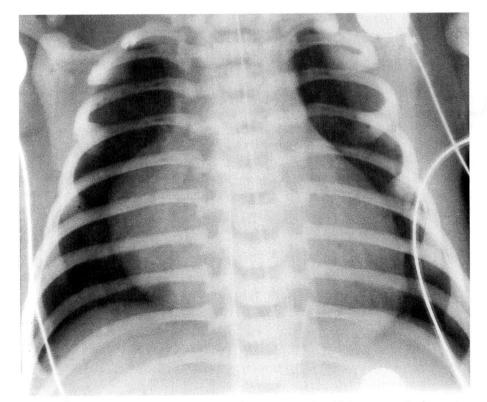

Figure 1-6   Right atrial enlargement in pulmonary atresia with intact ventricular septum. This patient had moderate tricuspid regurgitation. Note the decreased vascularity in the lungs.

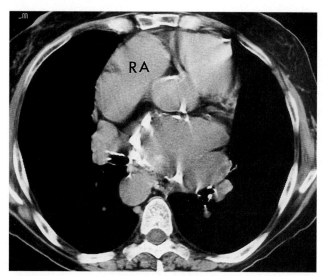

Figure 1-7   Right atrial enlargement in rheumatic heart disease. The appendage portion of the right atrium (RA) touches the anterior chest wall in this patient, who had a sternotomy for mitral valve replacement. The right coronary artery is visible in the fat between the right atrium and right ventricle. The left atrium is calcified and also enlarged.

Left Atrium

There are many clues to left atrial enlargement on the frontal and lateral chest film. One of the earliest signs of slight enlargement is the appearance of the double density, which is the right side of the left atrium as it pushes into the adjacent lung. Because a prominent pulmonary vein or varix may also cause a vertical double density, for the double density to present it should begin to curve inferiorly (Figure 1-10). In extreme cases, the left atrium may enlarge to the right side and touch the right thoracic wall (Figure 1-11). The etiology of this "giant left atrium" is rheumatic heart disease, mainly from mitral regurgitation.

A convex left atrial appendage on the frontal view is abnormal and usually reflects prior rheumatic heart disease. In pure mitral regurgitation, the body of the left atrium, but not the appendage, enlarges.

The following indirect signs are visible only when the left atrium is dilated at least moderately (Box 1-4, Figures 1-12, 1-13).

Common acquired causes of left atrial enlargement are mitral stenosis or regurgitation, left ventricular failure, and left atrial myxoma. Congenital causes include ventricular septal defects, patent ductus arteriosus, and the hypoplastic left heart complex. When atrial fibrillation occurs, the left atrial volume may increase by 20%.

Left Ventricle

Left ventricular enlargement exists if the left heart border is displaced leftward, inferiorly, or posteriorly. Inferior

---

Box 1-4   Left Atrial Enlargement on Chest Film

Convex left atrial appendage
Double density on the left side as the left atrium extends into the left lower lobe
Posterior displacement of the barium filled esophagus
Displacement of the left main stem bronchus posteriorly on the lateral view and superiorly on the frontal view (Figure 1-13)
Spreading of the carina

---

displacement may invert the diaphragm and cause this border to appear in the gastric air bubble. The chest film cannot reliably distinguish between left ventricular dilatation and hypertrophy. With hypertrophy, the apex has a pronounced rounding and a decrease in its radius of curvature. The elderly normal heart also has this shape. When massive hypertrophy is present, the left ventricular shape is large and appears similar to one that is only dilated (Box 1-5).

Common causes of left ventricular enlargement can be grouped into three categories: pressure overload (hypertension, aortic stenosis; Figure 1-14); volume overload (aortic or mitral regurgitation, ventricular septal defects; Figure 1-15); and wall abnormalities (left ventricular aneurysm, hypertrophic cardiomyopathy; Figure 1-16).

CARDIAC AND PERICARDIAL CALCIFICATIONS

Calcium in the heart is not only a marker for specific diseases but also an aid for locating structures on the chest film. Structures that calcify usually can be located easily on routine frontal and lateral films, although, in special situations, oblique views with barium may be necessary. Most of the calcium found in the heart is dystrophic and is in tissue that has had a previous inflammatory process (e.g., rheumatic mitral stenosis) or has been in a malformed structure that has degenerated (e.g., bicuspid aortic valve).

Box 1-5   Left Ventricular Enlargement on Chest Film

Rounding of the cardiac apex
Enlargement to the left, inferior or posterior

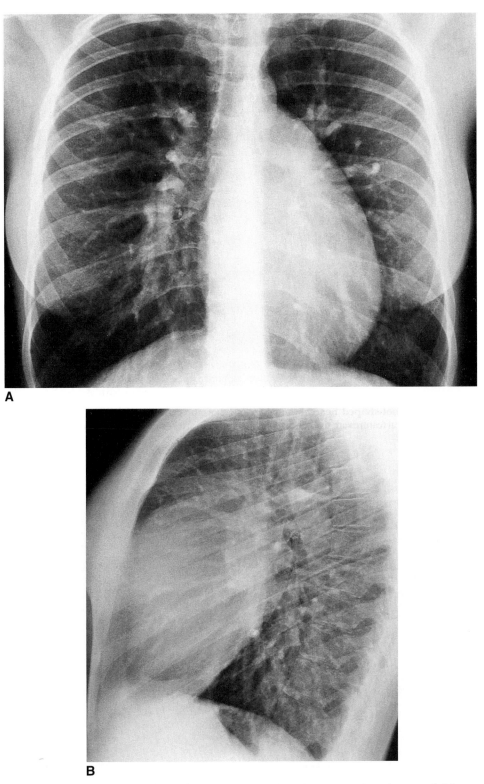

Figure 1-8   Right ventricular enlargement. A, The broad convexity along the upper left heart border represents the dilated right ventricle. **B,** The right ventricle touches the sternum and fills one-third of the retrosternal space. Shunt vascularity is also evident in this patient with atrial septal defect.

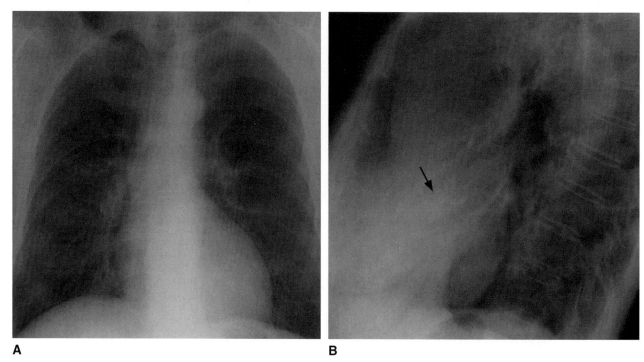

A   **B**

Figure 1-14   Aortic stenosis. A, The left ventricle is enlarged to the left and inferiorly where it is seen through the stomach bubble. The ascending aorta has poststenotic dilatation. **B,** The posterior border of the left ventricle is significantly behind the inferior vena cava. Note moderate calcium in the aortic valve (arrow).

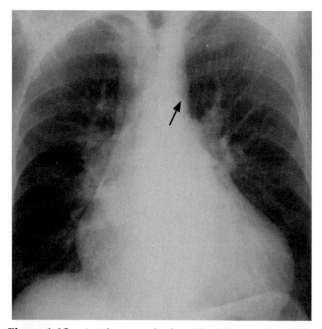

Figure 1-15   Aortic regurgitation. The left ventricle and the aorta are both large from moderate aortic regurgitation. The indentation in the descending thoracic aorta (arrow) and the absence of rib notching denote a pseudocoarctation. Because 50% of those with pseudocoarctation have a bicuspid aortic valve, this probably is the etiology of the aortic regurgitation.

Aortic Valve Calcification

Distinguishing Characteristics

Calcium in the aortic valve is seen best in the lateral view, where it projects free of the spine. You can distinguish between aortic and mitral calcification by the following methods.

- If the ascending aorta is dilated, follow its curvature back to locate the aortic valve in the middle of the cardiac silhouette.

- On the lateral view, if you draw a line from the junction of the diaphragm and the sternum to the carina, it will pass through the aortic valve (unless the thoracic cage is quite distorted or there is severe right heart enlargement). The mitral valve lies posterior to this line (Figure 1-17).

- Aortic calcification may have a specific appearance. Calcification in a bicuspid aortic valve, which never occurs before age 35, is dystrophic and involves the raphe and edges of the cusps. The calcification is linear in the raphe and may curve along the cusp edge. A nearly circular calcification with an interior linear bar in the aortic region is diagnostic of a bicuspid valve (Figure 1-18). In older patients with bicuspid aortic stenosis, this architecture is obliterated by nodular masses of calcium; in this instance the severely calcified aortic valve looks identical to that of the three major causes of aortic stenosis:

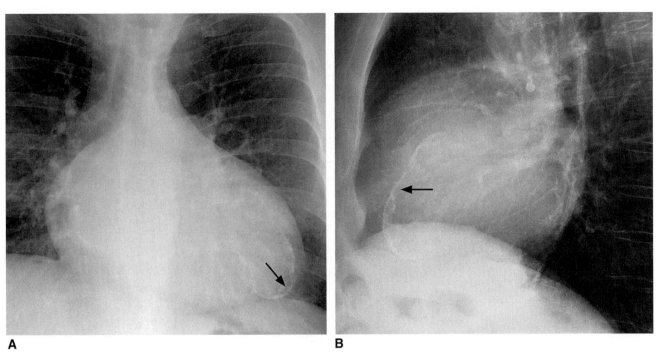

A   **B**

Figure 1-16   Left ventricular aneurysm. This angular left ventricular border with curvilinear calcification (arrow) is characteristic of an aneurysm.

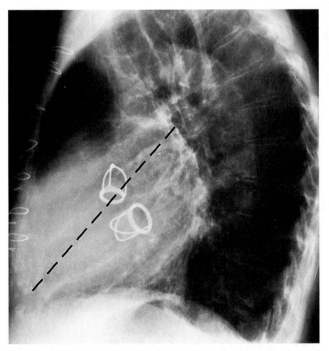

Figure 1-17   Location of the aortic valve on the lateral chest film. A line drawn from the junction of the diaphragm and the sternum to the carina passes through the aortic valve. The mitral valve is below and posterior.

bicuspid valve, rheumatic heart disease, and degenerative calcific aortic stenosis.

Calcific Aortic Stenosis

Calcium in the aortic valve may extend from the valve into the adjacent interventricular septum and cause arrhythmias. In most cases of bicuspid aortic stenosis, the mitral valve is normal and the left atrium is not enlarged. When both the aortic and mitral valves are calcified, the cause is usually rheumatic heart disease. In a patient without rheumatic heart disease or a previous episode of infected endocarditis, calcification in a tricuspid aortic valve is rare before age 70. Patients with bicuspid aortic valves also may have had rheumatic heart disease or endocarditis and develop heavy central calcification.

The aortic valve is the only one that has a good correlation between the amount of calcium seen on a chest film and the amount of stenosis. If the patient is over age 35, heavy calcification in the aortic valve indicates severe stenosis that will probably require a valve replacement. Conversely, if no calcium is seen by fluoroscopy in the aortic valve, it is unlikely that aortic stenosis exists.

Mitral Annulus Calcification

Distinguishing Patterns

The mitral valve ring may calcify in individuals over age 60. The incidence is four times higher in women.

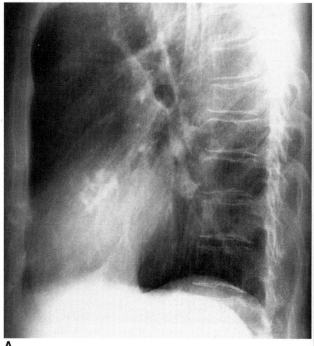

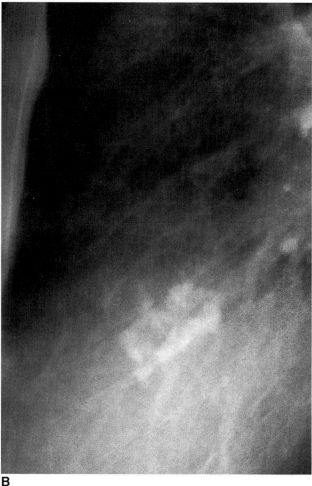

A

B

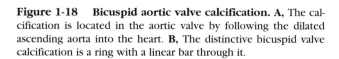

Figure 1-18   Bicuspid aortic valve calcification. A, The calcification is located in the aortic valve by following the dilated ascending aorta into the heart. **B,** The distinctive bicuspid valve calcification is a ring with a linear bar through it.

The calcium begins to form in or below the mitral annulus at the junction between the ventricular myocardium and the posterior mitral leaflet. More severe degrees of calcification will form a pattern resembling the letter J, the letter O, or a reversed letter C (Figure 1-19). In extreme cases, the mass of calcification can grow posteriorly into the ventricular myocardium to produce heart block. It can also grow anteriorly into the leaflets of the mitral valve to cause mitral regurgitation and stenosis. Rarely, the calcification can erode through the endocardium and cause small systemic emboli. Mitral annulus calcification in the elderly is associated with a doubled risk of stroke, independent of the traditional risk factors.

Clinical Significance
In most instances, mitral annulus calcification has little clinical significance and is a noninflammatory chronic degenerative process. Aortic stenosis and hypertension have a higher incidence of mitral annulus calcification, possibly because of increased strain exerted on the mitral valve apparatus from the left ventricular pressure overload. For the same reason, the tricuspid annulus rarely may calcify when right ventricular pressures have been chronically increased (Figure 1-20).

Mitral Valve Calcification

Causes
Mitral leaflet calcification is almost always caused by chronic rheumatic valvular disease. Rarely, the leaflets are calcified from infected endocarditis or from tumors attached to the mitral valve. There is limited correlation between the hemodynamic severity of mitral stenosis and the amount of calcium in the valve. Although a severely calcified mitral valve is usually stenotic, mitral stenosis frequently exists with no calcium in the valve.

Appearance
Radiologically, the calcium first appears as fine speckled opacities and later coalesces into larger, amorphous masses (Figure 1-21).

As the rheumatic valvulitis progresses, causing commissural fusion, chordal shortening, and fibrosis, the leaflet calcification may extend into the chordae and to the tip of the papillary muscles. Tricuspid calcification from rheumatic valvulitis is rare, and pulmonary calcification from rheumatic heart disease does not occur.

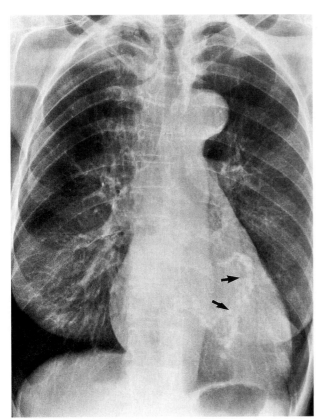

Figure 1-19 Mitral annulus calcification. The characteristic oval calcification (arrows) is located below the left atrial appendage segment.

Myocardial Calcification

A myocardial infarction can later calcify if it evolves to form either a scar or an aneurysm. You will easily recognize the thin curvilinear calcification as it projects within the left ventricular wall and inside the heart silhouette (Figure 1-22).

Occasionally, the tip of an infarcted papillary muscle will calcify; the ensuing mitral regurgitation represents papillary muscle dysfunction. The anterolateral, apical, and septal walls of the left ventricle are the usual locations for true aneurysms and therefore are the typical locations for myocardial calcification.

Left Atrial Calcification

Left atrial calcification is the sequela of rheumatic endocarditis. The appearance usually is curvilinear around the body of the left atrium (Figure 1-23). The interatrial septum does not calcify but the appendage does, and has a shaggy nodular appearance. The calcium deposits may be shaggy but usually occur in an "eggshell" pattern (Figure 1-24). Left atrial wall calcification indicates that the patient is in atrial fibrillation. Mural thrombi over the calcium are frequently present and may embolize into

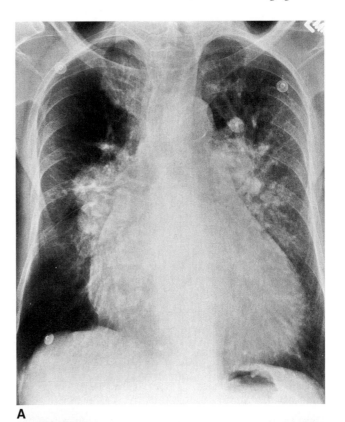

A

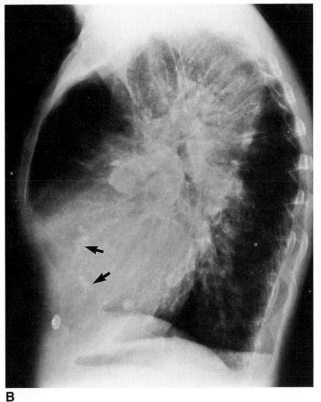

B

Figure 1-20 Tricuspid annulus calcification. A, Adult tetralogy of Fallot with unusually large mediastinal collaterals to the pulmonary hila. **B,** The tricuspid annulus (arrows) calcified because of the chronic right ventricular hypertension.

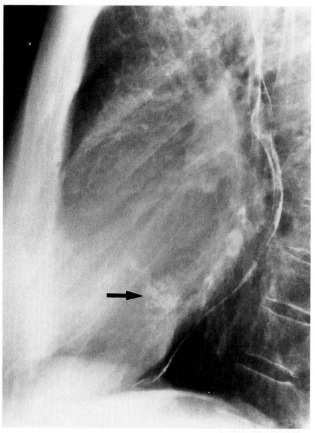

Figure 1-21   Calcified mitral valve. The barium-filled esophagus is displaced posteriorly around the large left atrium. The mitral valve (arrow) is heavily calcified.

the systemic circuit. Tumors in the left atrium, such as myxomas, calcify with an incidence of less than 5%.

Pericardial Calcification

Causes
Calcific deposits in the pericardium represent the end stage of a nonspecific inflammatory process. Tuberculosis, viruses and many other infectious agents, rheumatic fever, uremia, and trauma all may cause local or diffuse calcification. Large localized masses of calcification suggest that the etiology was tuberculosis.

Radiologic Appearance
The calcification radiologically appears in two forms:
- clumpy amorphous deposits, frequently in the atrioventricular grooves
- diffuse eggshell calcification involving most of the cardiac silhouette, except the left atrium, which is not covered with pericardium (Figure 1-25).

Use of Computed Tomography
In patients with constrictive pericarditis, 50% have calcium visible on the chest film, and most have calcium on the CT scan. Because pressure tracings from the ventricles may be identical in both restrictive cardiomyopathy and constrictive pericarditis, a CT scan that shows calcium in a thickened pericardium in a patient with elevated filling pressure is diagnostic of constrictive pericarditis (Figure 1-26).

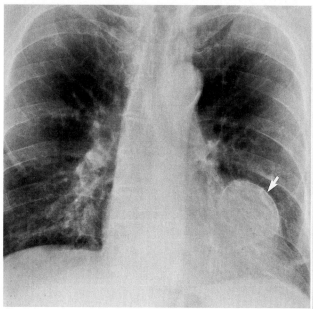

A

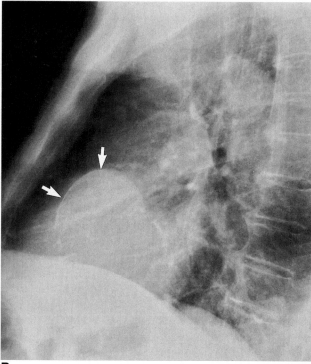

B

Figure 1-22   Calcified left ventricular aneurysm. The rim of calcium (arrows) outlines a saccular aneurysm in the anterolateral wall.

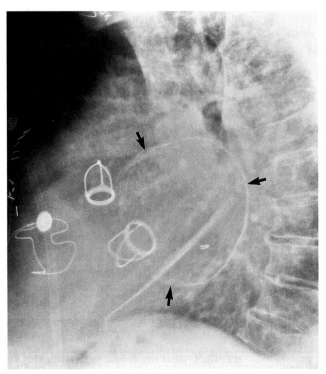

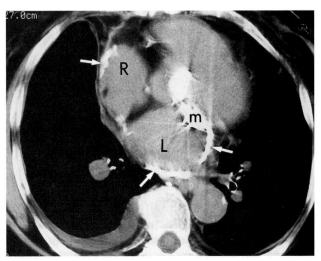

Figure 1-24   Right and left atrial calcification. Linear nodular calcification (arrows) is present in the right atrium (R) and left atrium (L) in this patient who had a mitral valve replacement (m).

Figure 1-23   Left atrial calcification. The large left atrium (arrows) has eggshell calcification extending superiorly to the left main stem bronchus and inferiorly to the mitral valve replacement. Aortic and tricuspid valve replacements are also present.

Coronary Calcification

Appearance

Coronary calcification represents atherosclerotic changes in the intima and in the internal elastic membrane of the coronary arteries. The left anterior descending artery is the most frequently calcified site, followed by

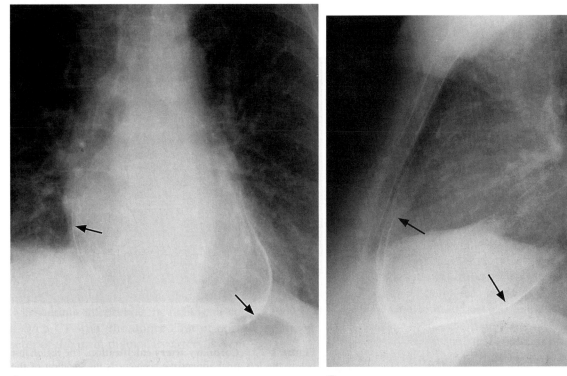

A   **B**

Figure 1-25   Pericardial calcification. A, Eggshell calcification (arrows) outlines the right and left borders of the heart. **B,** Diffuse calcification projects over most of the heart and reflects circumferential deposits.

Box 1-6 Examples of Decreased Pulmonary Vasculature

Congenitally Hypoplastic Pulmonary Arteries

By location
- Diffuse hypoplasia
- Segmental stenoses
- Main pulmonary artery (supravalvular pulmonary stenosis)
- Bifurcation of right and left pulmonary artery
- Branch or peripheral pulmonary arteries

By disease
- Williams syndrome
- Noonan syndrome
- Ehlers–Danlos syndrome
- Cutis laxa
- Alagille syndrome (biliary hypoplasia and vertebral anomalies)

Complex anomalies with right-to-left shunts
- Tetralogy of Fallot
- Pulmonary valve atresia with or without a ventricular septal defect
- Ebstein's anomaly

Acquired Small Pulmonary Arteries

Central obstruction
- Emboli
- Tumor

Hilar
- Takayasu's disease
- Rubella
- Emboli

Precapillary obstruction
- Air trapping diseases such as emphysema and Swyer–James syndrome

---

can be used as a standard. Peripheral pulmonary emboli; congenital branch stenosis; Takayasu's disease; and destruction of a lung by previous pneumonia, abscess, or bulla all may have caused decreased pulmonary vasculature in only a single lobe. Pulmonary stenosis with any malformation that allows a right-to-left cardiac shunt can cause diminished flow to the lungs. For example, patients with tetralogy of Fallot have decreased pulmonary vasculature because of the pulmonary stenosis and right-to-left shunt across the ventricular septal defect. Box 1-7 gives examples of decreased pulmonary vasculature.

High-output States

Segmental Analysis

The size of the central, hilar, and peripheral pulmonary arteries and veins reflects in a complex way the pressure, flow, and volume in the lungs. In a high-output state, all pulmonary segments are enlarged: the central pulmonary artery segment is convex, the hilum appears engorged, and the peripheral vessels are large from apex to base.

Flow Ratios

High-output states can be separated into those that have increased blood flow in both the pulmonary and the systemic circulation and those that have increased pulmonary circulation only. The chest film usually does not detect increased pulmonary flow until the flow ratio ($\dot{Q}_P/\dot{Q}_S$) is at least 2, i.e., the pulmonary flow is twice that in the aorta. Increased cardiac output from both the right and left ventricles occurs in metabolic and endocrine diseases, in arteriovenous fistulas and malformations, and in aortic regurgitation.

Contributing Diseases, Lesions, and Defects

Thyrotoxicosis (Figure 1-30), beriberi, and pheochromocytoma are diseases that either increase the overall metabolic rate of the body or have a specific effect on the heart. They increase its rate and stroke volume. Extracardial shunts such as patent ductus arteriosus, aortopulmonary window, and arteriovenous fistulas and malformations either in the lungs or in another part of the body provide a lower-resistance parallel circuit to the systemic capillary bed for the blood to return to the heart. (The electrical analogy is a short circuit of a battery, which causes a high current to flow across its terminals.) In Paget's disease there are numerous arteriolar–venous channels within the bone. In aortic regurgitation, blood flow that is regurgitated from the aorta into the left ventricle is added to the forward output to produce an augmented forward flow in the aorta. Because the lungs are in a series circuit with the aorta, the output is also increased. Intracardiac shunts have a normal aortic size and large main, hilar, and peripheral pulmonary arteries. In babies, high-output states often result in an element of pulmonary edema (Figure 1-31). A large pulmonary vasculature is also a feature of certain cyanotic congenital heart diseases (Figure 1-32).

A convex main pulmonary artery segment suggesting a high-output state may be present in healthy individuals. Highly trained endurance athletes, such as marathon runners, women in the third trimester of pregnancy, and occasionally teenage girls frequently show mild enlargement of the main pulmonary artery (Box 1-7).

Pulmonary Artery Hypertension

Pressure Measurements and Patterns of Pulmonary Vasculature

Pulmonary hypertension exists when the pulmonary systolic pressure is greater than 30 mmHg and the mean pressure exceeds 20 mmHg. Pulmonary hypertension

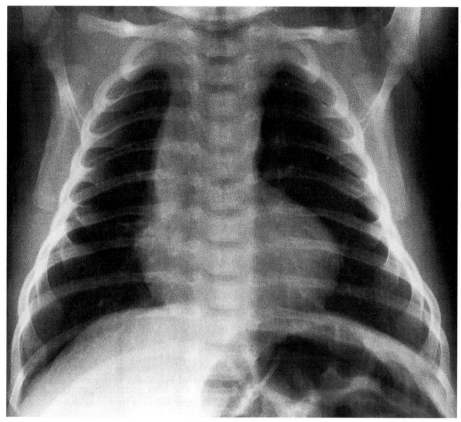

Figure 1-29   Decreased pulmonary vasculature. The main pulmonary artery segment is concave, the hilar arteries are small, and the peripheral vessels are indistinct in this patient with tetralogy of Fallot.

---

may occur when there is increased resistance in any part of the pulmonary circulation from the pulmonary artery to the left heart. The type of pattern of the pulmonary vasculature on the chest film depends upon the location of the abnormal resistance, the chronicity, and the severity.

If the heart is structurally intact, the earliest sign of pulmonary artery hypertension is a convex main pulmonary artery segment. Severe, chronic pulmonary artery hypertension also dilates the hilar branches but, unlike a left-to-right shunt, not the peripheral arteries within the lungs (Figure 1-33). The gradient of small vessels at the apex and large vessels at the base is preserved.

Eisenmenger Syndrome

In adults with Eisenmenger syndrome the pulmonary vasculature is unusually striking because of the central arterial enlargement. The arteries dilate longitudinally, forming a serpentine course (Figure 1-34). The rapid taper of the large aneurysmal hilar pulmonary arteries to the periphery looks like a "pruned tree." This phrase is correct angiographically and pathologically: there are fewer arterial side branches than in a normal arterial tree. However, the reduced number of side branches can not

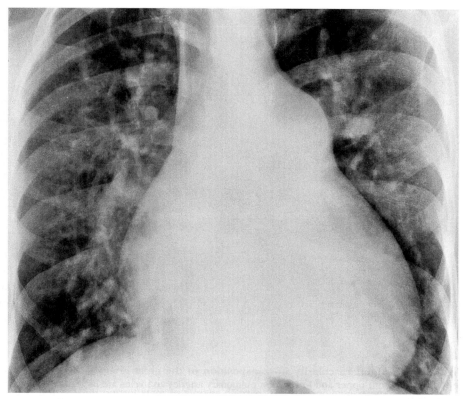

Figure 1-34   Eisenmenger syndrome. In addition to the large main pulmonary artery segment and hilar branches, the peripheral pulmonary arteries are large and have a serpentine course.

be seen on a chest film. The size of the pulmonary arteries in relation to their adjacent bronchus is measurable on CT (Figure 1-35).

Box 1-8 lists the common causes of pulmonary artery hypertension.

Venous Hypertension

The pulmonary pattern in pulmonary artery hypertension that is secondary to pulmonary venous hypertension has a different time course and appearance. After weeks to months of increased pulmonary venous pressure,

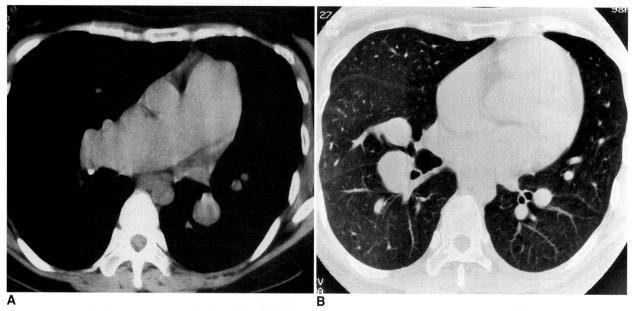

A   **B**

Figure 1-35   CT scan of pulmonary artery hypertension. A, The diameters of the main and right pulmonary arteries are almost twice that of the adjacent aorta. **B,** The hilar pulmonary arteries are two to three times larger than their adjacent bronchus.

Box 1-8   Common Causes of Pulmonary Artery Hypertension

Obstruction in the Central Pulmonary Arteries

Thromboembolism or tumor
Peripheral pulmonary stenosis
Hypoplastic pulmonary arteries

Increased Resistance in the Capillary Bed

Obstructive or interstitial lung disease
Widespread airspace disease such as pneumonia,
    tumor, atelectasis, or pneumonectomy
Primary pulmonary hypertension
Eisenmenger syndrome

Obstruction to Pulmonary Venous Drainage

Left ventricular failure
Restrictive cardiomyopathy such as amyloid
Mitral stenosis (Figure 1-36)
Hypoplastic left heart syndrome
Pulmonary veno-occlusive disease
Fibrosing mediastinitis

the hilar and central segments of the pulmonary arteries begin to dilate. The peripheral pulmonary branches continue to suggest pulmonary venous hypertension with large vessels at the apex and small vessels at the lung base.

Pulmonary Venous Hypertension

Pulmonary edema – excessive fluid in the alveolar and interstitial compartments of the lung – has two clinical classifications: cardiogenic and noncardiogenic. Cardiogenic edema is caused by pulmonary venous hypertension and is most commonly the result of left ventricular failure or acute mitral regurgitation. In the infant, it may result from hypoplastic left heart syndrome or total anomalous pulmonary venous connection below the diaphragm.

Noncardiogenic or permeability edema is the accumulation of fluid in the lungs in the presence of normal left atrial pressures. This has many complex causes that disrupt the alveolar capillary membrane.

Fluid and Water Exchange

Pulmonary edema has many radiologic patterns and, to analyze these more exactly, it is important to have an

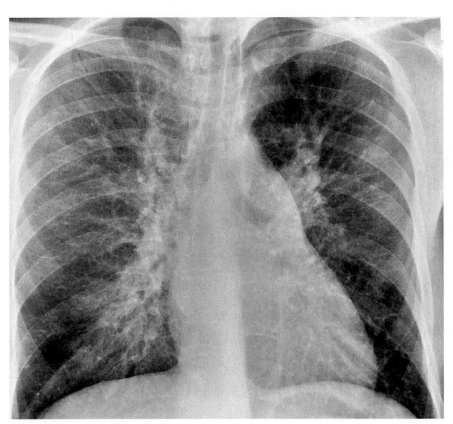

Figure 1-36   Pulmonary artery hypertension from mitral stenosis. The central pulmonary artery is convex and the hilar arteries are large because of arterial hypertension. The large upper lobe pulmonary arteries and veins and invisible lower lobe vessels indicate pulmonary venous hypertension. Note the double density along the right side of the heart from left atrial enlargement.

understanding of lung architecture and physiology for gas and fluid exchange.

In the normal lung, hydrostatic and osmotic forces provide a gradient to keep fluid within the pulmonary microvasculature. Fluid exchange mainly takes place across the alveolar–capillary endothelium as well as the interstitium around the precapillary and postcapillary vessels. The alveolar septum is differentiated into one side with thin cells for gas exchange and one side with thick cells for fluid exchange. When interstitial pulmonary edema develops, the water and protein accumulate predominantly on the thick side.

The lung removes excess fluid mainly by a network of pulmonary lymphatics. The mediastinal and pulmonary

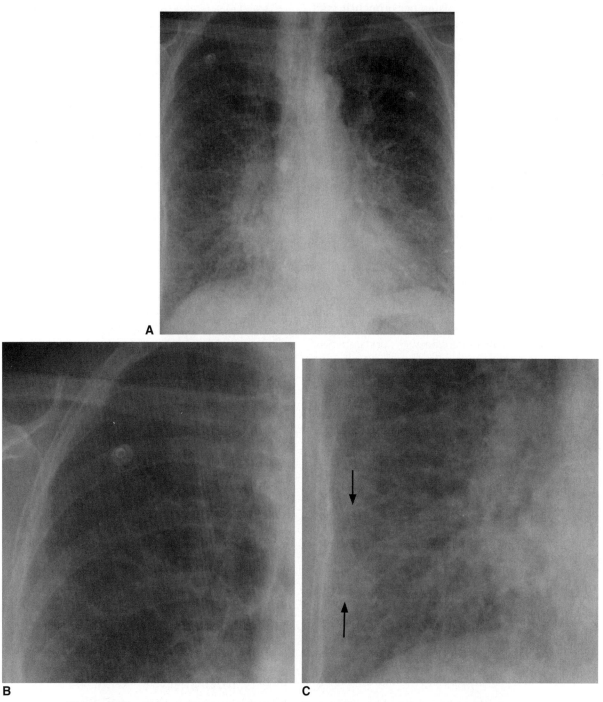

Figure 1-37   Pulmonary venous hypertension. A, The upper lobe arteries and veins are dilated out to the cortex and are the same size as the lower lobe vessels. **B,** The dilated upper lobe arteries are larger than their adjacent bronchus. Many more vessels are now visible. **C,** The lower lobe arteries and veins are indistinct. Several Kerley B lines (arrows) are visible in the subpleural space.

lymphatics serve as the major channel for fluid removal. Extensive lymphatic channels exist near the alveolar ducts and drain centrally adjacent to respiratory bronchioles, to the interstitium about the minor and major bronchi, and to the major mediastinal lymph nodes. The cortex of the lung has its own lymphatic supply, which drains the peripheral portion of the lung into pleural lymphatics. This anatomic arrangement provides a pathologic correlation that explains peribronchial cuffing and hilar haze on the chest film as two signs of pulmonary edema. When there is significant accumulation of lung water, the rate of lymph flow can increase tenfold before there is significant pulmonary edema. The excess lung fluid in the pulmonary interstitium is visible in patients with transplanted lungs because the lymphatics have been cut, blocking the major pathway of fluid transport from the lung.

Radiologic Appearance
The radiologic appearance of pulmonary venous hypertension with the later formation of pulmonary edema has a distinct time course and appearance that frequently separates it from other types of diffuse lung disease and noncardiogenic pulmonary edema. As the left atrial pressure rises from its normal value of less than 12 mmHg, the size of the pulmonary veins changes and fluid begins to appear in the interstitium. The first two signs to appear on the upright chest film are that the lower lobe vessels become indistinct and the upper lobe vessels begin to dilate. In normal appearance of the lower lobe vasculature, vessel edges are sharp, multiple secondary branches are clearly visible, and the average size of vessels in the middle part of the lung between the hilum and cortex is 4–8 mm. At least five to eight arteries can be seen at the right base. This effect is predominantly due to gravity in the upright person, giving greater blood flow and blood volume to the lower lobes.

As left atrial pressure rises, the hilar and lower lobe vasculature becomes indistinct and the edges are less sharp. Fluid begins to accumulate in the interstitium. The number of visible side branches decreases, perhaps because of a silhouette sign as water in the interstitium partially obscures the adjacent vessel wall. In response to the higher venous pressure, the upper lobe vessels handle the blood that is meeting increasing resistance as it enters the left atrium. You will recognize this increased blood flow to the upper lobes by the increased visibility of numerous upper lobe arteries and veins (Figure 1-37). The width of these structures, normally 1–2 mm in the middle part of the lung, increases to 2–4 mm. The redistribution now is reflected by an increase in both the size and number of vessels in the apices. The development of pulmonary venous hypertension is a continuum in the gradient of vessel size from apex to base. The normal distribution of small apical and large basilar vessels becomes balanced with equal size in both locations; at higher pressures this reverses and the upper lobe vessels are larger. A CT scan of a supine person with pulmonary venous hypertension will show large anterior vessels and smaller posterior vessels. Roughly the same branching generation from the main pulmonary artery should be used when comparing the anterior and posterior arteries (Figure 1-38).

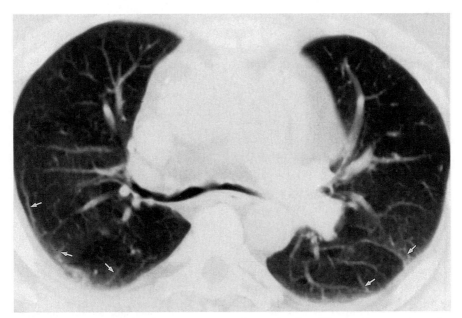

Figure 1-38   CT scan of pulmonary venous hypertension. The anterior vessels are larger than the corresponding posterior vessels in this supine scan. Kerley B lines are adjacent to the right lung pleura posteriorly and a linear subpleural opacity in the posterior left lung (arrows).

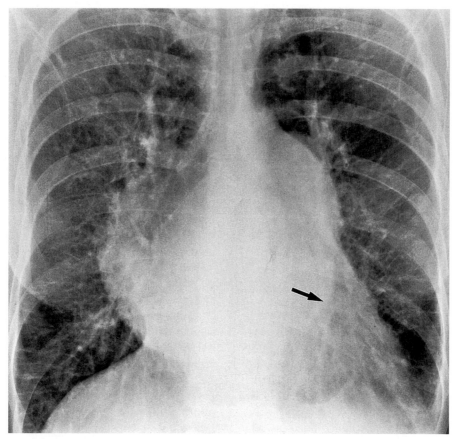

Figure 1-39   Kerley B lines. Bilateral linear opacities in the costophrenic sulci represent distended interlobar septa. These lines may extend along the lateral wall nearly to the apex. Mitral stenosis has enlarged the left atrium and distorted the right side of the heart. A double density (arrow) along the left heart border is the interface of the large left atrium with the lung. The convex main pulmonary artery indicates pulmonary artery hypertension.

There are other signs of interstitial lung water that help confirm the diagnosis of pulmonary venous hypertension. In the cortex of the lung, Kerley B lines appear and represent thickening of the interlobular septum (Figure 1-39). Kerley A lines – 3–5 cm lines about 1 mm thick and extending from the central part of the lung – represent distended lymphatics (Figure 1-40). The perihilar haze probably represents a combination of distended lymphatics, alveolar transudate, and interstitial thickening in lung parenchyma that lies anterior and posterior to the hilum. Thickening of the interlobular fissures and accumulation of subpleural fluid represent excess fluid and distention of the interstitial space and lymphatics. The end-on appearance of the bronchus and its adjacent pulmonary artery also changes in pulmonary venous hypertension. The bronchial wall becomes thickened and less distinct ("cuffed") and the pulmonary artery dilates (Figure 1-41).

As interstitial edema proceeds to alveolar edema, roseate opacities begin to appear in the perihilar region and spread peripherally to form a "butterfly pattern." This does not involve the lung cortex except in extreme cases.

When the opacities involve a significant part of the lung cortex and its adjacent pleura, other disease processes, such as pneumonia and adult respiratory distress syndrome, are more likely explanations for the cortical distribution. The edema caused by a cardiac disease typically is symmetrical and perihilar and is more severe in the lung bases than in the apices. The distribution of cardiac pulmonary edema can be quite variable and asymmetric but is never completely unilateral. Asymmetric pulmonary edema is usually more severe in the right lung. These patients are often lying with their right side down so the distribution of pulmonary edema often corresponds to the gravity gradient. Patients who develop mitral regurgitation during myocardial infarction rarely may also have pulmonary edema, predominantly in the right upper lobe. The jet of mitral regurgitation is directed into the right upper pulmonary vein and augments the forces in that lung that promote fluid retention.

Pleural and pericardial effusions develop in patients with left heart failure. In edema, the subpleural interstitial pressure rises sufficiently to create a net pressure into the pleural space. Generally, the pulmonary venous

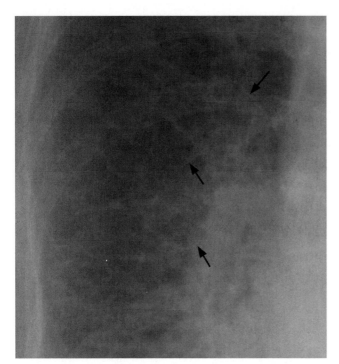

Figure 1-40   Kerley A lines. Central linear opacities (arrows) that are perihilar and do not conform with fissures are distended lymphatics.

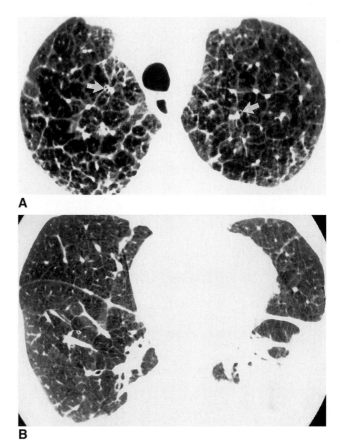

A

B

Figure 1-41   High-resolution CT of cardiac interstitial edema. A, The secondary pulmonary lobules are outlined by the thickened interstitium in this patient with emphysema. The bronchovascular bundles (arrows) have a pulmonary artery larger than the adjacent bronchus. **B,** A basal section shows thickening of the major fissures with dependent posterior pleural effusions. The secondary lobules are visible because of a thickened interlobar septum. The bronchial walls are thickened, which is the plain chest film correlate of "cuffing."

pressure needs to exceed 20 mmHg to have visible pleural effusions. Isolated elevation of pulmonary arterial pressure does not produce pleural effusions.

The width of the vascular pedicle is an indirect but reliable sign of increased intravascular fluid. The width is measured just above the aortic arch from the left subclavian artery on the left side to the superior vena cava on the right side (Figure 1-42). Dilatation of this pedicle and the adjacent azygos vein is increased in overhydration, renal failure, and chronic cardiac failure. In contrast, the vascular pedicle is usually unchanged in capillary permeability edema.

The time course of the appearance and disappearance of pulmonary edema on the chest film is variable but, in slowly progressing clinical situations, there is a rough correlation with the pulmonary capillary wedge pressure. When the wedge pressure is greater than 20 mmHg, there are always detectable signs of pulmonary venous hypertension and pulmonary edema on the chest film.

There is only a fair correlation between redistribution of blood flow with dilatation of the upper lobe vessels and pulmonary capillary pressure between 12 and 20 mmHg. Because the osmotic pressure of plasma protein is 25 mmHg, it is reasonable to expect alveolar edema when the pulmonary capillary wedge pressure exceeds this number; however, alveolar opacities can be seen with pressures of only 20 mmHg. Pulmonary edema

may be visible within a few minutes after the onset of acute mitral regurgitation or left heart failure. As the pulmonary edema resolves, there may be a therapeutic lag during which the wedge pressure returns to normal while the pulmonary edema persists. This lag may exist from several hours to several days. Although it is common to compare interpretation of the pulmonary edema on the chest film with the pulmonary capillary wedge pressure, these two observations measure different parameters and therefore are not appropriate standards of comparison. The pulmonary capillary wedge pressure measures the instantaneous pulmonary venous and left atrial pressures. The radiologic signs of pulmonary edema are an integrated history of the production and resorption of lung water. Particularly in the resorption phase, these signs more accurately mirror the amount of lung water present rather than the pulmonary venous pressure. A patient with an acute myocardial

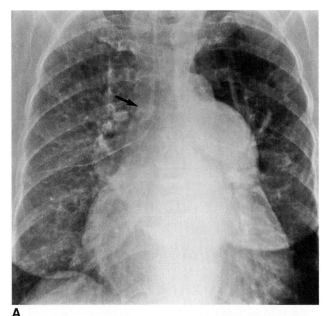

A

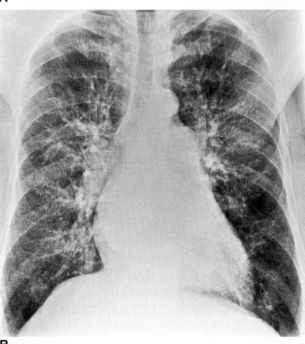

B

Figure 1-42   Width of the vascular pedicle as an indicator of fluid status. A, The wide vascular pedicle measured above the aortic arch reflects a dilated superior vena cava. The azygos vein (arrow) is also large. **B,** This patient also has pulmonary edema but a small vascular pedicle, probably reflecting vigorous diuretic therapy that reduced the intravascular volume. The residual pulmonary edema represents a therapeutic time lag.

infarction who has a chest film showing pulmonary edema and a normal pulmonary wedge pressure has stiff and noncompliant lungs because of the unresorbed interstitial fluid.

Box 1-9 lists the cardiac causes of pulmonary edema.

<hr />

Box 1-9   Cardiac Causes for Pulmonary Edema

Obstruction

At pulmonary vein level
- Congenital pulmonary vein atresia
- Pulmonary veno-occlusive disease
- Extrinsic pulmonary vein obstruction by tumor or fibrosing mediastinitis
- Total anomalous pulmonary venous connection below the diaphragm

At left atrial level
- Cor triatriatum
- Left atrial myxoma or tumor
- Left atrial thrombus

At mitral valve level
- Mitral stenosis or regurgitation

At left ventricular level
- Left ventricular infarct, aneurysm, or failure
- Hypoplastic left heart syndrome
- Cardiomyopathy with stiff left ventricular walls
- Left coronary artery from the pulmonary artery

At aortic valve level
- Aortic stenosis (valvular, subvalvular or supravalvular)

At aorta level
- Hypoplastic aorta
- Coarctation
- Takayasu aortitis

High-output Failure

Systemic vasodilation (septic shock)
Mitral or aortic regurgitation
Thyrotoxicosis
Large ventricular septal defect
Patent ductus arteriosus
Peripheral arteriovenous fistula

<hr />

SKELETAL ABNORMALITIES IN HEART DISEASE

Cardiac Surgery

The appearance of the thoracic cage can indicate previous surgery and frequently suggests certain types of heart disease. Most cardiac surgery begins with a median sternotomy because it gives excellent access to the heart's anterior structures and to the ascending aorta. A sternotomy also causes less postoperative pain than a posterior thoracotomy. After many types of cardiac surgery, there may be sternal wire sutures, mediastinal clips, epicardial pacing wires, and umbrella closure devices (Figure 1-43). A myriad of vascular clips following the course of the left internal mammary artery indicates a graft to the left anterior descending or diagonal

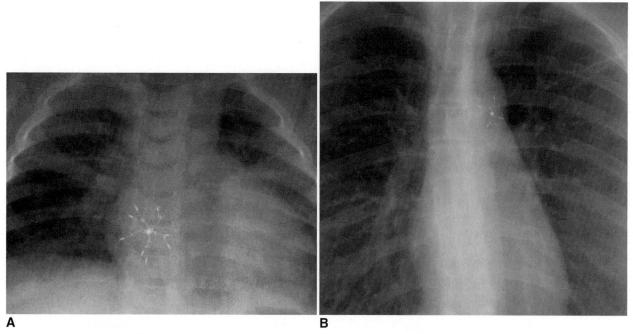

A   **B**

Figure 1-43   Umbrella closure devices. A, For an atrial septal defect. **B,** For a patent ductus arteriosus.

arteries. Most prosthetic mitral and aortic valve replacements are easily seen (Figure 1-44), except for the St Jude valve, whose ring is usually not visible. The leaflets of this valve appear as one or two straight lines and are seen in about 30% of chest films when the leaflets are tangential to the x-ray beam. You can identify a posterior thoracotomy by a surgical absence of the fifth rib or by uneven spacing between the fourth, fifth, and sixth ribs. Left posterior thoracotomies are performed to repair a coarctation of the aorta, to ligate a patent ductus

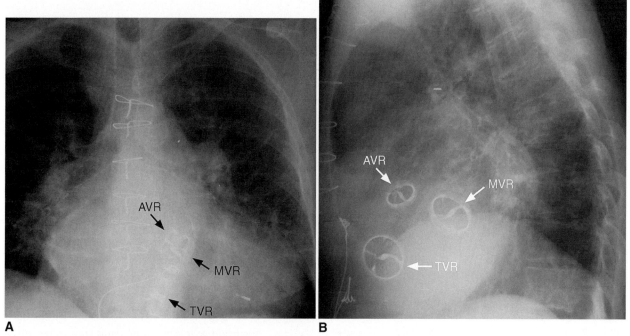

A   **B**

Figure 1-44   Mechanical prosthetic valves. Mechanical prosthetic valves in the aortic (AVR), mitral (MVR), and tricuspid (TVR) positions. On the frontal view (**A**), the valves tend to overlap each other. The lateral view (**B**) separates the valves and allows a subjective measurement of the size of the adjacent chamber.

arteriosus, to repair a vascular ring, and to create a left Blalock–Taussig shunt between the left subclavian artery and the left pulmonary artery. Right posterior thoracotomies are performed to create a right Blalock–Taussig shunt or to approach a coarctation in the right aortic arch.

Thoracic Cage and Heart Disease

The thoracic cage also has several distinctive signs associated with heart disease. The chest film of a patient with Marfan syndrome may show a tall person with a narrow anteroposterior diameter and a pectus excavatum (Figure 1-45). However, a normal variation is a narrow posteroanterior diameter of the thorax, which has a structurally normal heart that is rotated to the left side. The lateral chest film then shows a straight thoracic spine lacking the normal kyphosis and diminished retrosternal and retrocardiac spaces. In the adult, when the distance between the sternum and the spine is less than 10 cm, the heart and mediastinum are shifted to the left side, producing an extrinsic levocardia.

Congenital Syndromes with Heart Disease

Spine abnormalities also may indicate surgery or disease. An acquired scoliosis may occur where the ribs on the side of a posterior thoracotomy have been pulled tightly together. Vertebral anomalies, such as hemivertebra and "butterfly" vertebra, are frequently associated with congenital heart disease (Figure 1-46).

Chest radiographs of infants with trisomy 21, or Down syndrome, may be distinctive enough to diagnose not only the heart disease but also the syndrome. Of patients with trisomy 21, roughly half have atrioventricular canal defects. Conversely, of those infants who have atrioventricular canal defects, about half have trisomy 21. Other indicative chest radiographic findings include 11 pairs of ribs (Figure 1-47) and multiple manubrial ossification centers (Figure 1-48), both of which are more prevalent in infants with trisomy 21 than in normal newborn infants.

The bony abnormalities in neurofibromatosis mimic the rib notching seen in coarctation of the aorta. The

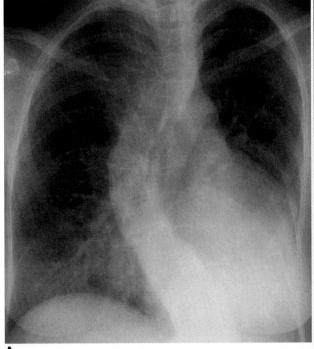

A

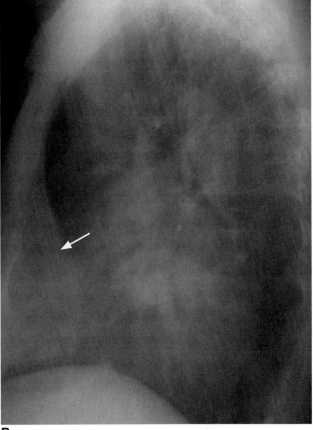

B

Figure 1-45   Marfan syndrome. A, The heart is shifted into the left hemithorax because of the severe scoliosis. The lungs have large volume. The aorta and the main pulmonary artery are dilated. **B,** The narrow anteroposterior diameter is accentuated by the pectus excavatum (arrow). The left ventricle is not enlarged but is rotated posteriorly by the skeletal deformity.

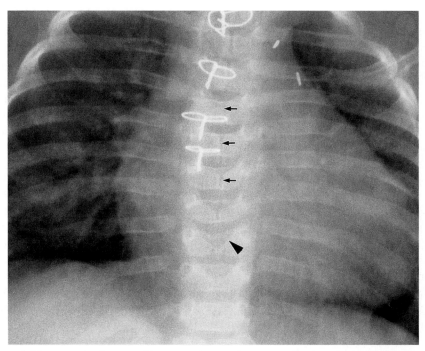

Figure 1-46   Vertebral anomalies. Butterfly vertebrae (arrowhead) and sagittal clefts (arrows) are associated nonspecifically with congenital heart disease. The large heart reflects left ventricular failure from the left coronary artery arising from the pulmonary artery.

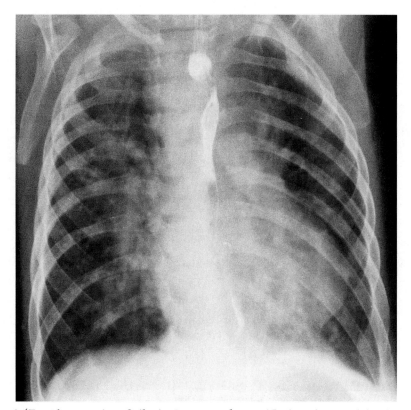

Figure 1-47   Eleven pairs of ribs in Down syndrome. The large heart and the shunt vascularity result from an atrioventricular canal defect. Barium in the esophagus is deviated by a right aortic arch.

also has large lobulated paravertebral masses of marrow hyperplasia and extramedullary hematopoiesis.

Many of the arthritic conditions are associated with fusiform aortic aneurysms, aortic regurgitation, and dissection. Ankylosing spondylitis, Reiter syndrome, and others may cause distinctive abnormalities in the spine. In ankylosing spondylitis, the apophyseal joints are fused and the posterior spinal ligaments are ossified. Syndesmophyte formation is recognized as a straight line or a smooth curve extending from the middle part of one vertebral body to the adjacent one. In contrast, the osteophytes that bridge the vertebral end plates denote degenerative spondylosis; this pattern has no association with heart disease.

Table 1-3 lists the major syndromes associated with cardiovascular disease.

THE CORONARY SINUS AND THE LEFT SUPERIOR VENA CAVA

Coronary Sinus

Anatomy and Relation to the Left Superior Vena Cava

The coronary sinus enters the right atrium anterior to the origin of the inferior vena cava. The eustachian valve of the inferior vena cava and the thebesian valve of the coronary sinus join to form a ridge of tissue between them. The coronary sinus extends behind the heart and becomes the great cardiac vein in the left atrioventricular groove. When a left superior vena cava is present, it joins the great cardiac vein about 2 cm from the right atrium to continue as the coronary sinus.

Table 1-3   Syndromes and metabolic disorders associated with heart disease

Cystic fibrosis	Cor pulmonale
DiGeorge syndrome	Aortic arch intrruption, truncus arteriosus, tetralogy of Fallot
Down sydrome	Endocardial cushion defect, mitral valve prolapse
Ellis-van Creveld syndrome	Atrial septal defect, single atrium
Ehlers-Danlos syndrome	Aortic aneurysms, dissection, and rupture; tortuous systemic and pulmonary arteries; congenital heart disease (valvular regurgitation and stenosis); mitral valve prolapse
Friedreich's ataxia	Hypertrophic cardiomyopathy
Homocystinuria	Marfan feature, coronary thrombosis
Mucopolysaccharidoses	Coronary artery disease, aortic and mitral stenosis and regurgitation
Osteogenesis imperfecta	Aortic regurgitation, aortic aneurysm
Progeria	Accelerated arteriosclerosis, hypertension
Sickle cell anemia	Cardiomyopathy, myocardial infarct, pulmonary infarct, cor pulmonale
Holt-Oram syndrome	Atrial septal defect, ventricular septal defect
Idiopathic hypertrophic subaortic stenosis	Hypertrophic cardiomyopathy, subaortic stenosis
Heterotaxy	Polysplenia or asplenia and congenital heart disease with anomalies of situs and symmetry
Ivemark syndrome	Asplenia and congenital heart disease with anomalies of situs and right-sided symmetry
Kartagener syndrome	Situs inversus with dextrocardia and bronchiectasis
Marfan syndrome	Aortic aneurysm/dissection; aortic, mitral, and tricuspid valve prolapse with regurgitation; mitral annular calcification in young adults
Neurofibromatosis	Aortic and pulmonary stenosis, pheochromocytoma with hypertension, coarctation, aortic aneurysm
Turner syndrome	Coarctation, aortic stenosis, atrial septal defect, pulmonary stenosis, aortic dissection
Noonan (male Turner) syndrome	Pulmonary valve and peripheral stenosis, atrial septal defect, idiopathic hypertrophic subaortic stenosis, ventricular septal defect, patent ductus arteriosus
Rubella	Peripheral and valvular pulmonary stenosis, patent ductus arteriosus, hypoplasia of the aorta, coarctation, atrial septal defect, ventricular septal defect
Treacher Collins syndrome	Atrial septal defect, patent ductus arteriosus, ventricular septal defect
Tuberous sclerosis	Myocardial rhabdomyoma
Williams syndrome	Supravalvular aortic stenosis, peripheral pulmonary stenosis

Data from Taybi H, Lachman RS: *Radiology of syndromes, metabolic disorders, and skeletal dysplasias,* ed 4, St Louis, 1996. Mosby–Year Book.

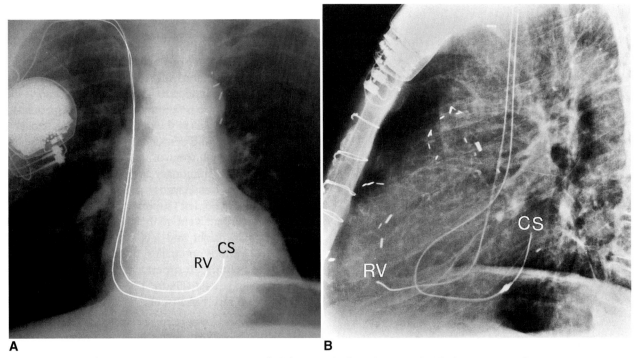

Figure 1-51   Coronary sinus and right ventricular wires. A, The dual pacing wires have a similar course on the frontal film. **B,** The lateral view separates the anterior right ventricular (RV) electrode from the posterior coronary sinus (CS) electrode.

Location from Catheter Position

On the frontal chest film a catheter ending in the coronary sinus usually cannot be distinguished from one ending in the body of the right ventricle. For this reason, you should use a lateral as well as a frontal view when placing a catheter or pacing wire into the right ventricle.

A power injection suitable for right ventriculography has enough force to rupture the coronary sinus into the pericardium. A lateral view identifies the posteriorly placed coronary sinus line from the right ventricular one (Figure 1-51).

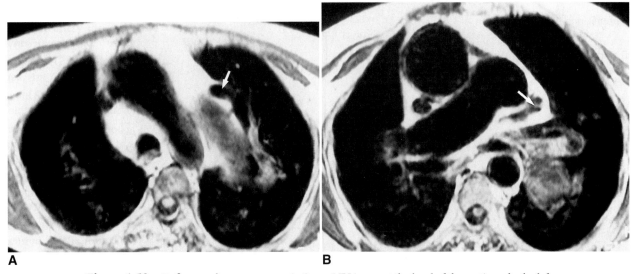

Figure 1-52   Left superior vena cava. A, On an MRI image at the level of the aortic arch, the left superior vena cava (arrow) is adjacent to the left pulmonary artery in this patient with truncus arteriosus. Although an anomalous pulmonary vein from the left lung may be in this position, lower slices (**B**) show its course (arrow) near the left pulmonary artery before it connects to the coronary sinus.

the chest wall, hyperinflated lungs, or pneumothorax. In infants and small children the subcostal window provides excellent images of all cardiac structures.

Suprasternal Imaging Planes

Suprasternal views are obtained by placing the transducer in the suprasternal notch. Both longitudinal and transverse planes of the great vessels can be imaged. The longitudinal plane orients through the long axis of the aorta and includes the innominate, left common carotid, and left subclavian arteries (Fig. 2-11). The transverse plane includes a cross-section through the ascending aorta, with the right pulmonary artery crossing behind. Portions of the innominate vein and superior vena cava are visible anterior to the aorta. The left atrium and pulmonary veins are posterior to the right pulmonary artery (Fig. 2-12).

Right Parasternal Views

The right parasternal border may also be useful for viewing the heart in either transverse or longitudinal orientations. These views are particularly helpful with medially positioned hearts, right ventricular enlargement, and rightward orientation of the ascending aorta. By allowing direct visualization of the right atrium, both venae cavae, and the interatrial septum, this view is also of particular value in the assessment of interatrial shunt flow, and in the detection of anomalous pulmonary venous drainage.

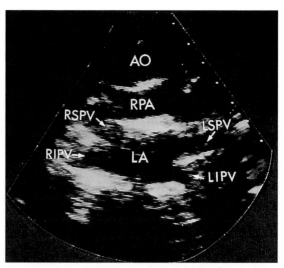

Figure 2-12   Two-dimensional suprasternal short-axis echocardiographic view of the aortic arch. The right pulmonary artery crosses beneath the aorta and the pulmonary veins enter the left atrium with a "crablike" appearance. Ao, aorta; LA, left atrium; LIPV, left inferior pulmonary vein; LSPV, left superior pulmonary vein; RIPV, right inferior pulmonary vein; RPA, right pulmonary artery; RSPV, right superior pulmonary vein.

Transesophageal Imaging

The esophagus is a valuable "window" to the heart and great vessels, especially in patients in whom transthoracic imaging is limited by either body habitus or lung disease. Further, transesophageal imaging is valuable in the operating room and intensive care setting, where it can help assess ventricular function or the adequacy of surgical repair of cardiac defects.

Transesophageal imaging uses a specially designed ultrasound probe incorporated within a standard gastroscope. This semi-invasive procedure requires blind esophageal intubation. Because of the close proximity of the heart to the imaging transducer, high-frequency transducers (5.0–7.5 MHz) are routinely used, which allows better definition of small structures than the lower frequencies used transthoracically (2.5–3.5 MHz). Therefore, transesophageal imaging is particularly valuable in the routine clinical setting for the detection of atrial thrombi, small vegetations, diseases of the aorta, and atrial septal defects, and the assessment of prosthetic valve function.

Current instrumentation allows imaging of multiple planes through the heart with multiplane transesophageal probes in which the ultrasound plane is electronically steered through an arc of 180°. The anteroposterior orientation of images from the esophagus is the reverse of images from the transthoracic window since the ultrasound beam first encounters the more posterior structures closest to the esophagus (Fig. 2-13).

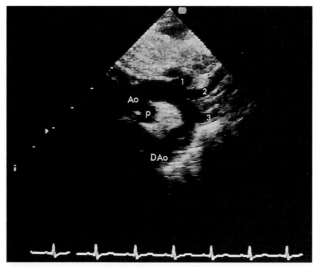

Figure 2-11   Two-dimensional suprasternal long-axis view of the aortic arch. The proximal portions of the brachiocephalic vessels are demonstrated arising from the aortic arch – (1) right brachiocephalic artery, (2) left common carotid artery, and (3) left subclavian artery. The right pulmonary artery can be seen in cross section as it passes beneath the ascending aorta. Ao, ascending aorta; DAo, descending aorta; p, right pulmonary artery.

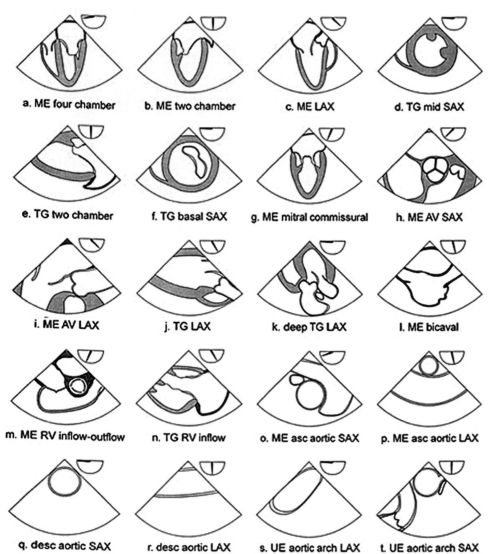

a. ME four chamber b. ME two chamber c. ME LAX d. TG mid SAX

e. TG two chamber f. TG basal SAX g. ME mitral commissural h. ME AV SAX

i. ME AV LAX j. TG LAX k. deep TG LAX l. ME bicaval

m. ME RV inflow-outflow n. TG RV inflow o. ME asc aortic SAX p. ME asc aortic LAX

q. desc aortic SAX r. desc aortic LAX s. UE aortic arch LAX t. UE aortic arch SAX

Figure 2-13 Diagrammatic representation of the standard imaging planes obtained with multiplane transesophageal echocardiography. Views from the upper esophageal, mid-esophageal and transgastric probe orientations are demonstrated. The approximate multiplane angle is indicated by the icon adjacent to each view. AV, aortic valve; LAX, long-axis; ME, mid-esophageal; RV, right ventricle; SAX, short-axis; TG, transgastric; UE, upper esophageal. (Reprinted with permission from Shanewise JS, Cheung AT, Aronson S, *et al.* ASE/SCA guidelines for performing a comprehensive intra-operative transesophageal echocardiographic exam. *J Am Soc Echocardiogr* 1991;12:887.)

THE NORMAL DOPPLER EXAMINATION

By applying the Doppler principle to ultrasound, you can analyze the frequency shift of ultrasound waves reflected from moving red blood cells to determine the velocity and direction of blood flow. This can be done with either pulsed Doppler or continuous wave Doppler. While pulsed Doppler allows analysis of the velocity and direction of blood flow at a specific site, continuous wave Doppler allows resolution and analysis of high-velocity flow along the entire length of the Doppler beam. In both instances the data can be displayed graphically (Fig. 2-14). By convention, flow toward the interrogating transducer is represented as a deflection above, and flow away from the transducer appears as a deflection below the baseline. The *x*-axis represents time and the *y*-axis represents velocity

calibrated in centimeters per second or meters per second.

Color-flow mapping also uses pulsed Doppler methodology but maps flow velocity at multiple sites within an area and overlays this information in color on a black-and-white two-dimensional image. By convention, color coding for flow velocity toward the transducer is red and flow velocity away from the transducer is blue. Higher velocities are mapped as brighter shades. The addition of yellow and green to the underlying red or blue color map indicates turbulent flow.

Parasternal Long-Axis View

In clinical practice, the routine Doppler examination is integrated with the sequence of imaging described above. Therefore, initial interrogation of the flow patterns associated with the aortic and mitral valves begins in the

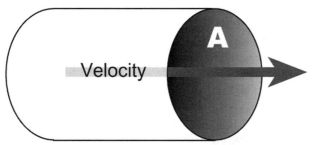

$$Flow(cm^3/min) = Area(cm^2) \times Velocity(cm/min)$$

Figure 2-35   Diagrammatic representation of the method for calculating cardiac output by the Doppler technique. Flow is the product of the velocity in centimeters per minute times the cross-sectional area through which the flow passes. This can be applied to flow across any of the cardiac valves but is most often used for the semilunar valves. The area is calculated by measuring the diameter (d) of the aortic or pulmonic annulus and assuming a circular cross-sectional area (A): $A = \pi(d/2)^2$.

area of the stenosis (A_2) if you know the velocity of flow through the stenotic region (V_2):

$$(V_1)(A_1) = (V_2)(A_2)$$

$$A_2 = \frac{(V_1)(A_1)}{(V_2)}$$

This concept allows calculation of the area of a stenotic valve (A_2):

- (V_1) = velocity of blood in the outflow tract determined by pulsed Doppler
- (A_1) = the area of the outflow tract calculated from the direct measurement of its diameter
- (V_2) = the peak velocity through the valve from the continuous wave Doppler profile across the stenotic valve.

Estimates of aortic valve area by this method relate reasonably well to those obtained from catheterization. However, they may be subject to error due to incomplete ascertainment of the maximal Doppler profile, the presence of atrial fibrillation, and errors in estimating the subaortic diameter.

Aortic Regurgitation

Until the addition of Doppler technology, echocardiography could only diagnose aortic regurgitation indirectly. High-frequency diastolic fluttering of one or both of the mitral leaflets suggests the presence of aortic regurgitation. Impingement of the regurgitant jet directly into the leaflets creates this echocardiographic finding. If regurgitation is severe, early diastolic closure of the mitral valve may occur.

Aortic valve abnormalities, such as a bicuspid valve or heavily calcified leaflets, raise the suspicion of associated valve regurgitation. Other morphologic features may indicate the cause of the regurgitant lesion. For example, leaflet prolapse may indicate the presence of a torn leaflet, and the presence of additional mobile echoes adherent to the valve may suggest endocarditis. Further, dilatation of the aortic sinuses or aortic root may indicate Marfan syndrome, ascending aortic aneurysm, or aortic root dissection.

As the severity of aortic regurgitation increases, the left ventricle dilates and hypertrophies. Systolic function is usually preserved until late in the course of the disease. Patients in whom the left ventricular systolic dimension reaches 55 mm tend to have a worse outcome following surgery. Indeed, there may be significant ventricular remodeling and restoration of systolic function following surgery.

Doppler techniques allow rapid detection of aortic regurgitation by color, pulsed, and continuous wave modalities (Fig. 2-36). In the parasternal long-axis views, aortic regurgitation appears by color Doppler as a diastolic red or blue jet emanating from the region of the aortic valve and directed into the left ventricular cavity. Sometimes the jet tracks along the anterior leaflet of the mitral valve. Parasternal short-axis views, as well as the apical five-chamber and apical long-axis views, may also allow detection of regurgitation, which appears as a red jet because it is directed toward the transducer.

Despite the ready detection of aortic regurgitation by color Doppler, assessing the severity of regurgitation is more difficult and at best only semiquantitative. For example, the use of jet length to assess the severity of regurgitation may be misleading as even small jets may coalesce with mitral inflow and appear large. An alternative is to consider the cross-sectional area of the jet in the short-axis plane or the jet width in the parasternal long-axis view; more severe regurgitation tends to fill a greater portion of the outflow tract in early diastole.

Pulsed Doppler can assess the severity of aortic regurgitation by detecting the presence of late diastolic flow reversal in the descending aorta, which invariably occurs with severe regurgitation. Finally, measurement of the regurgitant pressure half-time derived from the continuous wave Doppler profile reflects the instantaneous pressure gradient between the aorta and the left ventricle. Therefore, more rapid pressure half-times reflect rapid increases in diastolic pressure within the left ventricle and more severe regurgitation (see Fig. 2-36). In general, a pressure half-time below 200 msec is indicative of severe aortic insufficiency; however, the utility of this method is limited by the effects of other factors, which may raise left ventricular diastolic pressure unrelated to the degree of aortic regurgitation.

Pulmonary Valve Disease

The pulmonary valve is best visualized in the parasternal short-axis plane, although subcostal views are also useful in children. Patients with rheumatic heart disease may

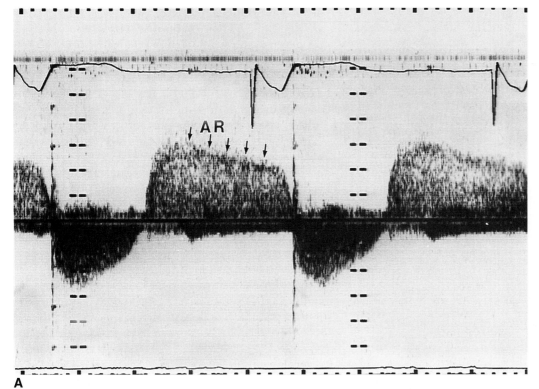

A

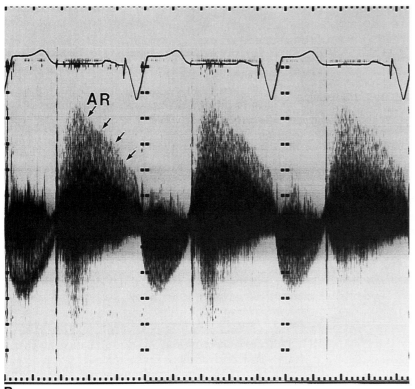

B

Figure 2-36 A, Continuous wave Doppler spectral trace in a patient with aortic insufficiency. The aortic flow is sampled from the apex with systolic outflow shown below the baseline and diastolic regurgitant flow above the baseline. With normal aortic and left ventricular diastolic pressures, the pressure difference between aorta and left ventricle remains high and the slope of the regurgitant velocities drops off gradually (arrows). In **B,** the aortic insufficiency is severe, causing a rapid equilibration of aortic and left ventricular diastolic pressures, resulting in a sharp slope in flow velocities (arrows).

have thickening of the pulmonary valve; however, significant pulmonary stenosis is rare. By far the most common cause of pulmonary stenosis is congenital deformity of the valve (Fig. 2-37). This may occur as a single lesion or in association with other defects (such as tetralogy of Fallot). Typically the valve appears mobile but the leaflets dome during systole. In routine practice continuous wave Doppler is used to assess the peak velocity across the valve, since this allows peak and mean transvalvular gradient calculation by the modified

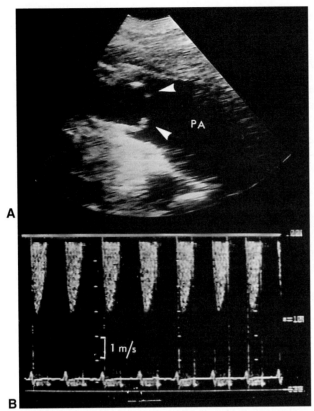

Figure 2-37 Two-dimensional image and continuous wave Doppler trace in a patient with valvular pulmonic stenosis. **A,** Parasternal long-axis echocardiographic view of the main pulmonary artery (PA). The leaflets are thickened and dome into the pulmonic root in systole (arrowheads). There is poststenotic dilatation of the main pulmonary artery. **B,** Doppler velocities across the valve show a peak systolic velocity of 3 m/sec, predicting a gradient of 36 mmHg. (From Liberthson RR. Congenital heart disease in the child, adolescent, and adult. In: Eagle KA, *et al.*, eds. *The practice of cardiology.* Boston, MA: Little, Brown, 1989.)

Bernoulli equation. There is often associated poststenotic dilatation of the proximal portion of the main pulmonary artery. Further, the right ventricle appears hypertrophied and the interventricular septum flattens during systole as a consequence of the increased pressure load.

Color Doppler commonly shows some degree of pulmonary regurgitation as a small red jet directed into the right ventricle toward the transducer. Small jets of regurgitation are physiologic. More marked degrees of regurgitation occur with pulmonary hypertension, primary valve disease, congenital absence of the pulmonary valve, or after pulmonary valvotomy. For clinical purposes, the degree of regurgitation is graded semiquantitatively, based on the width and length of the regurgitant jet.

Prosthetic Heart Valves

Prosthetic heart valves may be either bioprosthetic or mechanical. Bioprosthetic valves may be heterografts from pig or bovine valves or pericardium, or homografts derived from human aorta or pulmonary artery. Some are supported by three struts that connect to a valve ring while others are strutless, using the native valve leaflets and annulus. Mechanical valve design is more diverse. Some older devices have a ball-in-cage design while others have either a single or double tilting disk. Because of the variable nature of these prostheses, it is usually possible to determine the specific type of prosthesis by echocardiography, especially since mechanical devices tend to be more reflective. For example, Starr–Edwards valves have a characteristic protrusion of the cage into the left ventricle or aorta, and a unique pattern of ball motion and forward flow around the valve. In contrast, disk valves have a much lower profile, and disk motion may be clearly evident. Finally, bioprosthetic valves are usually recognizable by the supporting strut and by the presence of leaflet motion within the prosthesis (Fig. 2-38).

Not surprisingly, two-dimensional and Doppler echocardiography is invaluable in the routine assessment of prosthetic valve function. It allows assessment of the stability of the device and of the degree of stenosis of the prosthesis. Further, echocardiography can also detect regurgitation through or around the valve, vegetation or thrombus within or around the prosthesis, and can assess ventricular function during the postoperative period. Poor seating of the prosthesis may occur as a consequence of paravalvular infection or wear of the sutures supporting the valve ring. As the valve seating becomes unstable, invariably there is some degree of paravalvular regurgitation. With this instability, the valve ring is seen to move independently through the cardiac cycle. Marked "rocking" of the prosthesis is a poor prognostic sign because it suggests that at least one-third of the valve ring has become unstable. Since infective endocarditis is the most common cause of destabilization, it is important to exclude the presence of paravalvular infection or abscess formation. Although this can occasionally be done from surface imaging, transesophageal imaging is more sensitive and specific.

Continuous wave Doppler can assess the gradient across the prosthesis in the same manner as for native valves. When assessing the significance of the Doppler gradient, however, it is important to bear in mind the following factors:

- The Doppler gradient may overestimate the catheter gradient across both the St Jude tilting disk and Starr–Edwards valves by up to 40%
- Each type of prosthesis has different flow profiles
- Smaller prostheses will have higher gradients than larger prostheses of the same type
- The gradient across an aortic prosthesis is critically dependent on ventricular function.

Therefore, in order to make a meaningful statement about the significance of the Doppler gradient across a prosthesis, it is important to consider the size, type, and

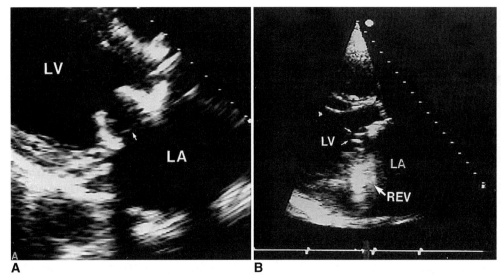

Figure 2-38   Parasternal long-axis echocardiographic view of the left heart in patients with prosthetic mitral valves. **A,** A bioprosthesis with echogenic struts protrudes from the mitral annulus into the left ventricle (LV). The bioprosthetic leaflets are thin and faintly seen within the struts (arrow). A St Jude tilting disk prosthesis is shown in **B**. Two parallel disks are shown in diastole (arrows). Dense reflections from the metallic structures of the valve appear as a bright reverberation (REV) in the left atrium (LA). (From Wilkins GT, *et al*. Echo-Doppler assessment of prosthetic heart valves. In: Weyman AE. *Principles and practice of echocardiography*, 2nd ed. Philadelphia, PA: Lea & Febiger, 1994.)

location of the prosthesis, as well as the left ventricular function.

Detection of a significant increase in gradient across a prosthesis is an important clinical sign because it may indicate valve occlusion or partial obstruction. This may be due either to pannus ingrowth around the sewing ring or to the presence of a large vegetation or thrombus within the valve apparatus.

To assess the significance of the degree of regurgitation across a prosthetic valve, it is important to consider the type and position of the prosthesis. The type of prosthesis is important since bioprosthetic and Starr–Edwards valves do not normally leak. In contrast, the single disk (Medtronic Hall) valve design allows a small central leak, and the double-disk St Jude valve has small leaks around the disk margins. Therefore, detection of a small central jet of regurgitation is expected in patients with disk valves, is suggestive of valve degeneration in a patient with a bioprosthetic valve, and may indicate either vegetation or pannus ingrowth around the valve ring in a patient with a Starr–Edwards valve (Fig. 2-39). Regardless of valve type, a paravalvular leak would indicate disruption of the valve ring due to either infection or wear of the valve sutures.

Assessment of the degree of regurgitation may be very difficult if not impossible in some patients because the reflectivity of the prosthetic material prevents sufficient penetration of the ultrasound signal beyond the prosthesis. This is particularly a problem in patients with both an aortic and a mitral valve prosthesis. Further, since the regurgitant jets tend to be eccentric, they are easy to miss during a routine examination. Although in some instances these problems can be overcome by imaging the heart in off-axis views, they can be completely overcome by using

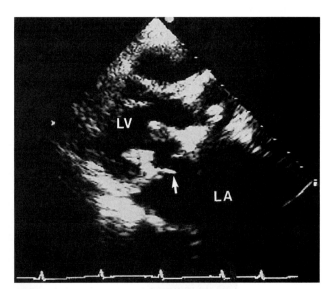

Figure 2-39   Parasternal long-axis echocardiographic view of the left ventricular inflow tract in a patient with a bioprosthetic mitral valve. The dense struts can be seen extending into the left ventricle (LV) from the annulus. The bioprosthetic leaflets have degenerated and one of the cusps is everted and prolapses into the left atrium (LA; arrow), creating severe mitral regurgitation. (From Wilkins GT, *et al.* Echo-Doppler assessment of prosthetic heart valves. In: Weyman AE. *Principles and practice of echocardiography*, 2nd ed. Philadelphia, PA: Lea & Febiger, 1994.)

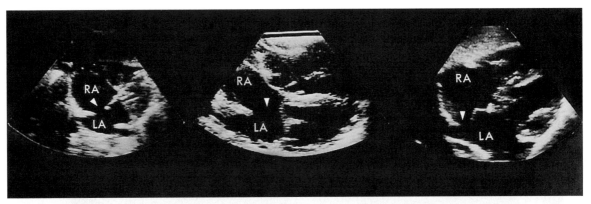

Figure 2-55 Subcostal echocardiographic views of the heart highlighting the interatrial septum. On the left, a defect in the midatrial septum represents a secundum atrial septal defect. The center panel demonstrates a large area of dropout from the mid-septum to the atrioventricular groove indicative of an ostium primum defect. In the panel on the right, a defect is present high in the atrial septum near the roof of the atria (arrowhead), consistent with a sinus venosus defect. LA, left atrium; RA, right atrium. (From Liberthson RR. Congenital heart disease in the child, adolescent, and adult. In: Eagle KA, *et al.*, eds. *The practice of cardiology*. Boston, MA: Little, Brown, 1989.)

Figure 2-56 Series of apical four-chamber echocardiographic views in a patient with an ostium primum atrial septal defect. In the upper left panel, the dropout in the lower atrial septum (arrow) delineates the defect. Doppler color flow mapping (upper right) demonstrates a wide band of flow crossing from the left atrium (LA) to the right atrium (RA; arrows). Following intravenous injection of agitated saline, microbubbles are detected as contrast within the cardiac chambers. In the lower left panel, right-to-left shunting can be seen across the defect (arrows) and left-to-right negative contrast is shown in the lower right panel (arrows) as unopacified blood crosses the atrial defect. LV, left ventricle; RV, right ventricle. (From Levine RA, *et al.* Echocardiography: principles and clinical applications. In: Eagle KA, *et al.*, eds. *The practice of cardiology*. Boston, MA: Little, Brown, 1989.) (See color inserts, Plate 5.)

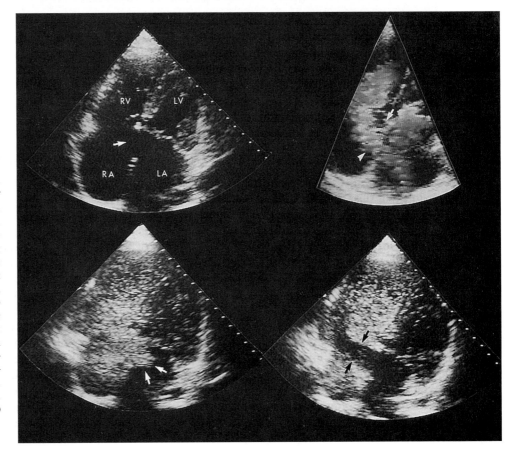

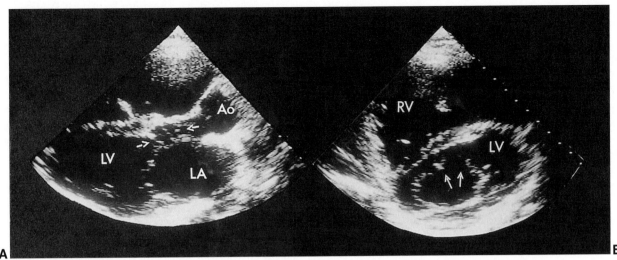

Figure 2-57   Parasternal echocardiographic views of the mitral valve in a patient with a partial atrioventricular canal defect. **A,** Chordal attachments of the anterior leaflet to the septum are seen (arrows). The cross-sectional view of the mitral valve (**B**) shows clearly the cleft in the anterior leaflet (arrows). Right ventricular enlargement and diastolic flattening of the interventricular septum are evidence of right ventricular volume overload from the associated atrial septal defect. Ao, aorta; LA, left atrium; LV, left ventricle; RV, right ventricle. (From King ME. Complex congenital heart disease II: a pathologic approach. In: Weyman AE. *Principles and practice of echocardiography*, 2nd ed. Philadelphia, PA: Lea & Febiger, 1994.)

chamber enlargement and paradoxical motion of the interventricular septum are indicative of right ventricular volume overload and generally indicate a pulmonary to systemic shunt ratio of greater than 1.5:1. Doppler estimates of volumetric flow across the pulmonic and aortic valves provides a noninvasive method of measuring the shunt ratio (see Fig. 2-19). The echo-derived shunt ratio ($\dot{Q}_p{:}\dot{Q}_s$) correlates well with that obtained at cardiac catheterization but is subject to measurement errors and therefore is used clinically only as a semiquantitative index of shunt size.

There are several methods for quantifying shunt flow by color Doppler, including measurements of the area of shunt flow within the right atrium and of the jet width as it crosses the defect. While the latter method correlates more closely with actual shunt size, both methods are still only semi-quantitative for clinical purposes.

The advent of percutaneous closure of ASD using a variety of devices has made definitive imaging of septal defect size, location, and number a clinical imperative. Because of the proximity of the source to the atrial septum from within the esophagus, transesophageal echocardiography is frequently used for a clearer image of atrial septal defects and to measure the size of the defect and its surrounding rims. Placement of the ASD closure devices in those defects that are amenable to percutaneous closure is accomplished in the cardiac catheterization laboratory under transesophageal echocardiographic guidance (Fig. 2-58). Transesophageal echo provides

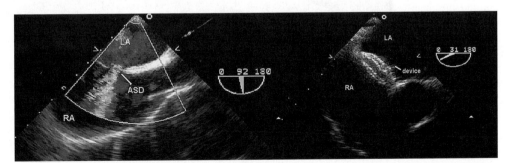

Figure 2-58   Transesophageal echocardiographic view of the interatrial septum. The panel on the left shows a discrete atrial septal defect (ASD) with color Doppler demonstration of shunting from left (LA) to right atrium (RA). The panel on the right shows a percutaneous closure device occluding the atrial septal defect (arrow). The device is well-aligned along the atrial septum with visualization of both the right and left atrial components. (See color inserts, Plate 6.)

preprocedural evaluation of the atrial septum, assists with catheter and sheath positioning, balloon sizing of the defect, and proper alignment of the device, and verifies device position and closure of the shunt following device deployment.

New technological advances have allowed the placement of ultrasound crystals on the tip of intracardiac catheters. These catheters can be positioned by the operator within the right atrium with the ultrasound image directed toward the atrial septum. Some centers now prefer to place ASD devices with guidance by intracardiac ultrasound instead of transesophageal imaging.

Ventricular Septal Defects

The interventricular septum is a complex structure composed of muscular and fibrous tissue. Defects in the septum are extremely common and can occur singly or multiply at many different locations. Figure 2-59 demonstrates the echocardiographic views in which each type of VSD can be recorded. Echocardiographic detection of a VSD depends on echo dropout from the interventricular septum and is further strengthened by the use of pulsed or color flow Doppler to detect turbulent shunt flow across the defect. Figure 2-60 shows representative echocardiographic examples of typical VSDs.

Muscular VSDs occur frequently in young children and the majority of these close spontaneously within the first 2 years of life. Muscular defects near the cardiac apex can be of considerable size and yet be overlooked unless the sonographer closely inspects the apical aspect of the interventricular septum.

The fibrous portion of the interventricular septum, the membranous septum, lies adjacent to the aortic annulus. Membranous septal defects cause septal dropout beneath the aortic valve. The tricuspid valve septal leaflet and chordal apparatus lie along the right ventricular aspect of the membranous septum. Incorporation of this tissue into a septal aneurysm often causes spontaneous closure of a membranous VSD. The right coronary or noncoronary aortic leaflet occasionally prolapses into a high membranous VSD, effecting defect closure but distorting aortic valve coaptation and causing aortic insufficiency (Fig. 2-61).

Supracristal VSDs occur in that portion of the interventricular septum located above the crista supraventricularis and beneath the pulmonary annulus. Echocardiographic views of the right ventricular outflow tract are best for detecting this type of defect. Prolapse and distortion of the right coronary aortic leaflet also occurs with supracristal VSDs.

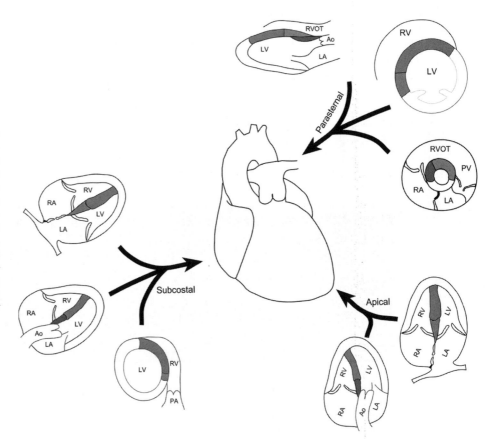

Figure 2-59 Diagrammatic representation of multiple echocardiographic views of the interventricular septum with variable shading of the subdivisions of the septum. The muscular septum, the inlet septum, the infundibular septum and the membranous septum are designated with variable shading (for fuller details, see color plate). Ao, aorta; LA, left atrium; LV, left ventricle; PA, pulmonary artery; PV, pulmonary valve; RA, right atrium; RV, right ventricle; RVOT, right ventricular outflow tract. (See color inserts, Plate 7.)

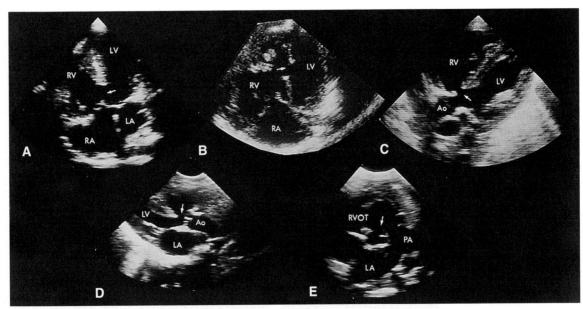

Figure 2-60   Series of echocardiographic views in patients with ventricular septal defects (VSDs; arrows). **A,** Apical four-chamber view of a complete atrioventricular canal. **B,** Apical four-chamber view of a muscular defect. **C,** Subcostal view of the left ventricular outflow tract with a membranous VSD. **D,** Parasternal long-axis view of a malalignment VSD with aortic overriding of the septum. **E,** Parasternal short-axis view of the aorta (Ao) with a supracristal defect. LA, left atrium; LV, left ventricle; PA, pulmonary artery; RA, right atrium; RV, right ventricle; RVOT, right ventricular outflow tract. (From Liberthson RR. Congenital heart disease in the child, adolescent, and adult. In: Eagle KA, *et al.*, eds. *The practice of cardiology*. Boston, MA: Little, Brown, 1989.)

Inlet VSDs occur in the region of the septum near the tricuspid and mitral annuli and are often associated with straddling of the tricuspid or mitral valves. Atrioventricular septal defects result from the absence of the atrioventricular septum and thus result in a large defect in the center of the heart that has an atrial and an inlet ventricular component. These are also known as "endocardial cushion" or "atrioventricular canal" defects.

When a VSD is restrictive in size and a significant pressure difference exists between left and right ventricles, pulsed and color flow Doppler readily detect the shunt flow across a VSD that may be too small to detect on two-dimensional imaging. A turbulent high-velocity jet enters the right side of the heart adjacent to the defect, and there may be flow within the septal tissue with acceleration along the left ventricular aspect of the communication (Fig. 2-62). When pressures equalize between left and right ventricles, shunt flow is low in velocity and thus may be difficult to discern by color flow mapping.

Echocardiography provides important clinical information on shunt size and pulmonary pressure. Significant left-to-right shunting through a VSD enlarges the pulmonary artery, left atrium, and left ventricle. Estimates of ($\dot{Q}_p$:$\dot{Q}_s$) can be made for shunts at the ventricular level, as described for atrial shunts. Using the simplified Bernoulli equation ($P = 4V^2$), the systolic pressure gradient between the left and right ventricles can be derived from the peak flow velocity of the left-to-right jet across the VSD. Subtracting this gradient from the aortic systolic blood pressure gives an estimate of the right ventricular and pulmonary artery systolic pressures.

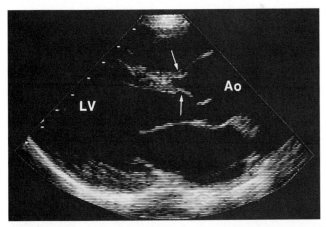

Figure 2-61   Parasternal long-axis echocardiographic view of the left ventricular outflow tract. The anterior cusp of the aortic valve has prolapsed into a high ventricular septal defect (arrows), effectively closing the interventricular communication but distorting the shape of the aortic valve creating aortic insufficiency. Ao, aorta, LV, left ventricle. (From Liberthson RR. Congenital heart disease in the child, adolescent, and adult. In: Eagle KA, *et al.*, eds. *The practice of cardiology*. Boston, MA: Little, Brown, 1989.)

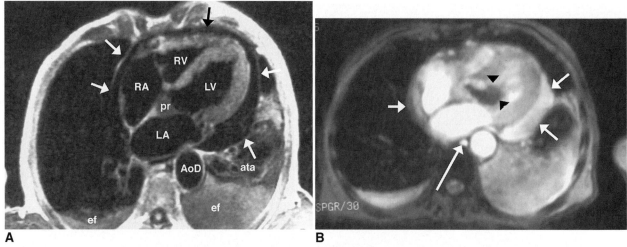

Figure 3-12   62-year-old man with severe acute aortic regurgitation. **A.** Axial double inversion recovery acquisition through the posterior right aortic sinus of Valsalva (pr). A large pericardial effusion surrounds the heart, separating the parietal pericardium (arrows) from the visceral layer. Notice the bilateral pleural effusions (ef) and left lower lobe atelectasis (ata). **B.** Gradient echo acquisition at the same anatomic level. The signal of the simple pericardial effusion is now bright (arrows). Also note the signal void of aortic regurgitation (arrow heads) extending from the aortic valve. The azygos vein (long arrow) is now a bright signal object as well. AoD, descending aorta; LA, left atrium; LV, left ventricle; RA, right atrium; RV, right ventricle.

ventricular function. The clinical and hemodynamic findings of constrictive pericarditis overlap with those of restrictive cardiomyopathy, a primary disorder of the myocardium. Differentiation between these two entities is imperative because patients with pericardial constriction may benefit from pericardiectomy; myocardial restriction may be rapidly progressive, and necessitate cardiac transplantation. Pericardial thickening is not diagnostic of pericardial constriction; demonstration of pericardial thickening greater than 4 mm (Figs. 3-15 and 3-17)

in face of characteristic hemodynamic findings distinguishes constrictive pericarditis from restrictive cardiomyopathy. Normal pericardium on MR is less than 4 mm in thickness.

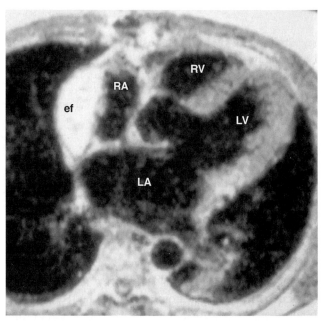

Figure 3-13   Axial double inversion recovery acquisition from a 30-year-old man who sustained sternal injury in a motor vehicle accident. The parietal pericardium (arrows) is separated by a predominantly high signal intensity material from the epicardial fat. Pericardial tap revealed blood. Notice the left pleural effusion (ef). Ao; aortic root; LA; left atrium; RA, right atrium.

Figure 3-14   Axial spin echo acquisition from a 60-year-old man with mild congestive heart failure. A high signal intensity loculated pericardial effusion (ef) subjacent to the pericardial fat and causing extrinsic compression of the right atrium (RA) slightly distorts the right heart border. The left atrium (LA), right (RV) and left (LV) ventricles are labeled.

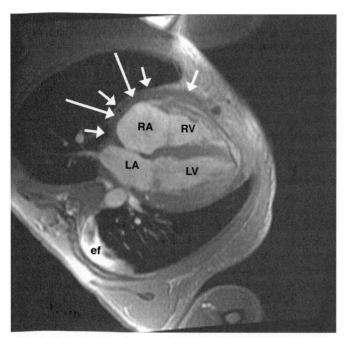

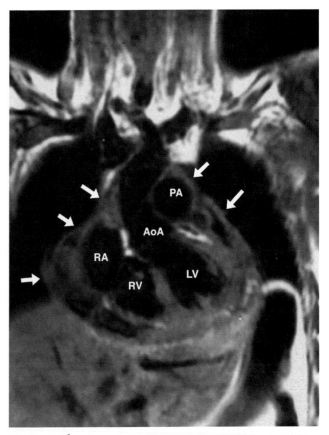

Figure 3-15   Diastolic four-chamber view gradient echo acquisition from a 32-year-old woman with progressive shortness of breath. The heart is nearly surrounded by an intermediate signal intensity band that is most apparent (short arrows) along the right atrial (RA) border. A faint bright signal (long arrows) within the intermediate signal represents free pericardial fluid between the thickened leaves of the pericardium. Notice the left pleural effusion (ef) and the increased distance between the chamber of the RA and the lateral heart border. LA, left atrium; LV, left ventricle; RV, right ventricle.

Figure 3-16   Coronal double inversion recovery acquisition from a 56-year-old man with chronic renal failure. The thickened, irregular pericardium (arrows) extends to the top of the main pulmonary artery (PA) along the left heart border, and along the right atrium (RA) and ascending aorta (AoA) on the right heart border. The pericardial space, i.e., the space beneath the cavities of the RA and RV, and below the left ventricle (LV), is increased in thickness, and filled with increased signal. Notice the overall globular appearance of the cardiac silhouette.

Magnetic resonance examination is exquisitely sensitive to changes in pericardial thickness, as well as to morphologic and functional changes in the atria and ventricles resulting from focal or diffuse pericardial disease. In pericardial constriction, the right ventricle may appear tubular in appearance. Gradient reversal acquisition demonstrates decreased right ventricular contractile function and limited diastolic excursion, common to both restriction and constriction. Dilatation of the right atrium, venae cavae, coronary sinus, and hepatic veins, reflecting right heart failure, may be found in cases of constrictive pericarditis as well as cases of restrictive cardiomyopathy (Fig. 3-18). However, in restrictive cardiomyopathy the pericardium is normal.

Calcium produces no magnetic resonance signal. Therefore, on spin echo MR, calcification appears as loci of irregular signal voids separating the epicardial and pericardial fat. In constrictive pericarditis, the circumcardiac signal void of the pericardial space is irregular.

Spin echo and gradient echo MR can also accurately evaluate the thickness of the posterior left ventricular wall in patients with constrictive pericarditis. Radiographic demonstration of thinning of the free wall of the left ventricle due to myocardial atrophy is associated with markedly increased mortality after pericardiectomy.

Pericardial Neoplasms

The wide field of view, excellent contrast resolution, and multiplanar capability of MR imaging make it a method of choice for diagnosis and evaluation of pericardial neoplasms. Pericardial effusion is the most common finding in patients with pericardial malignancy. Hemorrhagic effusion, frequently associated with primary malignant mesotheliomas, may present as areas of high, low, and medium signal intensity, depending on the age of the hemorrhage. Focal or generalized pericardial thickening may also be found in patients with malignant pericardial involvement. Direct invasion can be inferred if the normally pencil-thin pericardium appears thickened or interrupted in close proximity to a neoplasm (Fig. 3-19).

Malignant pericardial neoplasms tend to be bulky, often septate, inhomogeneous in signal intensity, and

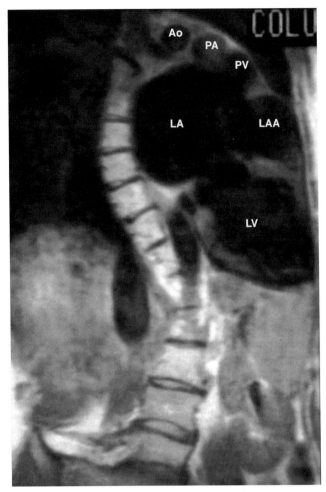

Figure 3-43 Coronal spin echo acquisition from a 34-year-old man with Marfan syndrome and mitral regurgitation. The markedly dilated left atrium (LA) and left atrial appendage (LAA), and dilated left ventricle (LV) are evident. Notice the dilated left upper lobe pulmonary vein (PV) as well. The distal main pulmonary artery (PA) appears greater in caliber than the distal aortic arch (Ao). The profound scoliosis is characteristic of patients with Marfan syndrome.

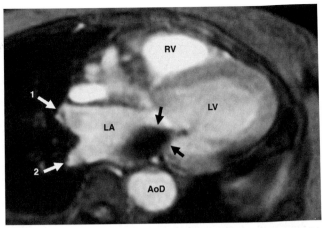

Figure 3-44 Axial early systolic oblique gradient echo acquisition from a 40-year-old man with chronic mitral regurgitation. The left ventricle (LV) and left atrium (LA) are both dilated. In addition, notice the dilated right upper (white arrow 1) and right lower lobe (white arrow 2) pulmonary veins. The right ventricle (RV) is normal. The signal void jet (black arrows) of the regurgitant flow extends from the mitral annulus into the LA.

Tricuspid regurgitation caused by pulmonary hypertension is associated with right heart and pulmonary artery dilatation. In these cases, spin echo and double inversion recovery pulse sequences reveal increased signal in the pulmonary artery segments caused by the slow blood flow and high pulmonary resistance (see Fig. 3-40). Left atrial enlargement and evidence of pulmonary hypertension in the face of a normal left ventricle point to mitral stenosis as a cause of the pulmonary hypertension and subsequent tricuspid dysfunction. Increased lung volumes and a normal left atrium suggest chronic obstructive pulmonary disease as the etiology. Patients with primary right heart failure will exhibit right heart dilatation, pleural and pericardial effusion, and evidence of right atrial hypertension, including dilatation of the inferior and superior venae cavae, coronary sinus, hepatic veins, and azygous vein. Finally, right heart enlargement with a small pulmonary artery indicates the decreased right ventricular output found in patients with Ebstein's anomaly. MRI provides unique insight into these causes of right ventricular disease.

Multivalvular Heart Disease

Valvular dysfunction is explicitly displayed using gradient echo acquisition as signal void jets. Recognizing the origin and direction of the jet, as well as the timing of the dysfunction, will clarify findings in patients with multivalvular heart disease. The most common etiology of multivalvular heart disease is chronic rheumatic heart disease. The most common combinations are mitral stenosis with aortic regurgitation, and mixed mitral and aortic regurgitation (Fig. 3-48).

Myocardial Tumors

Cardiac tumors are rare. Three-quarters of all primary tumors of the heart are benign, and of soft tissue origin: rhabdomyoma, fibroma (Fig. 3-49), lipoma, angioma, and myxoma. These tumors generally appear as infiltrating masses with signal intensity characteristic of the tissue of origin, i.e., high signal lipoma and intermediate signal intensity rhabdomyoma. Differentiation of these benign masses from their sarcomatous counterparts can be inferred by identification of a high signal intensity necrotic core, or other evidence of

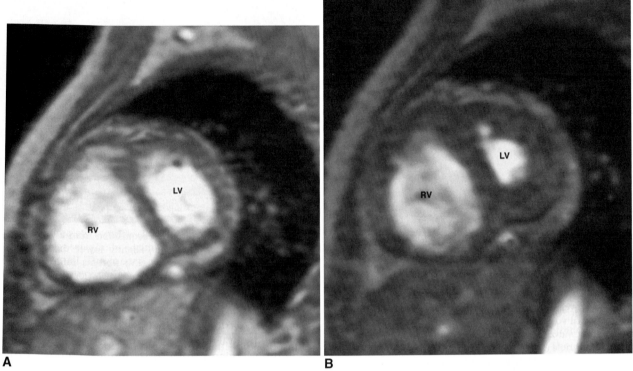

A   **B**

Figure 3-45   Short-axis gradient echo acquisition through the mid-heart from a 39-year-old man with primary pulmonary hypertension. **A.** End-diastolic image shows dilatation of the right ventricle (RV) with straightening of the interventricular septum. **B.** End-systolic image shows thickening of both the right (RV) and left (LV) ventricular myocardium, and straightening of the interventricular septum.

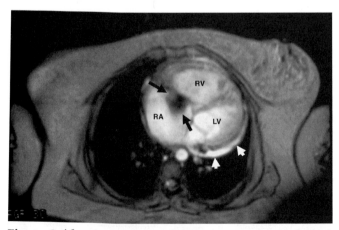

Figure 3-46   Axial systolic gradient echo acquisition from a 24-year-old woman with primary pulmonary hypertension. The free wall right ventricular (RV) myocardium is hypertrophied. The heart is rotated toward the left and the interventricular septum is nearly in the coronal plane. The broad signal void jet (black arrows) of tricuspid regurgitation extends into the dilated right atrium (RA). Notice the small pericardial effusion (white arrows).

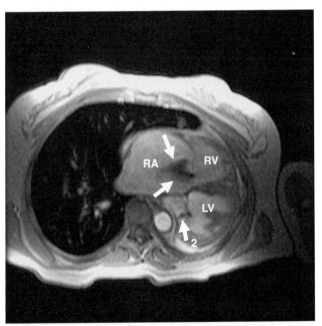

Figure 3-47   Axial early systolic gradient echo acquisition from a 24-year-old woman with pulmonary hypertension and agenesis of the left pulmonary artery. The heart is markedly rotated into the left chest. The right ventricular myocardium is moderately hypertrophied. The signal void jet of tricuspid regurgitation (arrows) extends into the dilated right atrium (RA). Also notice the dilated left ventricle (LV) and small jet (arrow 2) of mitral regurgitation. At this anatomic level, the enlargement of the left atrium cannot be appreciated.

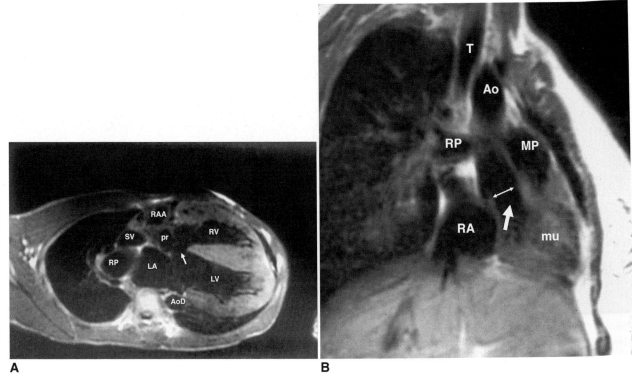

Figure 3-80   Two patients with subaortic (membranous) ventricular septal defect. **A.** Oblique axial double inversion recovery acquisition through the posterior right aortic sinus of Valsalva (pr) in a 25-year-old man with a large ventricular septal defect (arrow) and heart failure. The right ventricular (RV) myocardium is thickened, and the cavity is dilated, as evidenced from the clockwise rotation of the heart into the left chest. The left ventricle (LV) and left atrium (LA) are dilated, as is the right pulmonary artery (RP). Right heart failure is revealed by dilatation of the right atrial appendage (RAA) and superior vena cava (SV). AoD, descending aorta. **B.** Right anterior oblique sagittal spin echo acquisition through the muscular interventricular septum from a 16-year-old boy with mild shortness of breath. The left-sided aortic arch (Ao) displaces the trachea (T) to the right. Immediately beneath the aortic valve annulus (double-headed arrow) and superior to the muscular interventricular septum (mu) is the signal void (arrow) of the membranous ventricular septal defect. The main (MP) and visualized right (RP) pulmonary arteries are dilated.

exclusion of focal pulmonary artery stenosis are goals of MR examination. The aorta is dilated in pulmonary atresia with ventricular septal defect as well as in tetralogy of Fallot. Systemic-to-pulmonary artery collaterals are usually found posterior to the trachea and main bronchi. Patency of palliative shunts may be assumed when no intraluminal signal is identified on spin echo examination.

In patients with tricuspid atresia, the anterior atrioventricular ring is replaced by fat, and no continuity between the right atrium and right ventricle is found (Fig. 3-85). The right atrium is usually enlarged and the right ventricle is usually smaller than normal. A large interatrial communication can usually be demonstrated (Fig. 3-86). Axial and sagittal acquisition demonstrates commonly associated lesions, including ventricular septal defect, pulmonary atresia, and the relationship between the great arteries, as well as complications of elevated systemic venous pressure such as mediastinal and pericardial venous collaterals. The results of surgical palliation by the Fontan operation may be demonstrated directly. In addition, application of velocity mapping techniques allows accurate assessment of conduit obstruction.

Univentricular Hearts

Univentricular heart is a compromise term adopted to avoid the controversy concerning naming hearts with rudimentary ventricular chambers and unusual atrioventricular connections. When the main chamber is morphologically

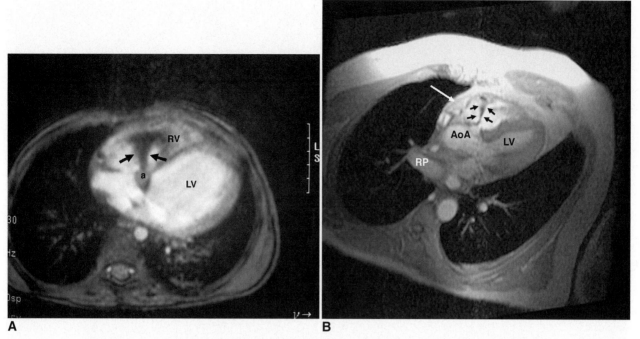

Figure 3-81   Two patients with ventricular septal defect. **A.** Axial systolic gradient echo acquisition from a 7-year-old boy. The right (RV) and left (LV) ventricles are dilated; the heart is rotated into the left chest. The fan-shaped signal void of the subaortic (membranous) ventricular septal defect (arrows) extends from just beneath the anterior aortic sinus of Valsalva (a), into the RV, and spreads in width as it strikes the RV free wall. **B.** Four-chamber view systolic gradient echo acquisition from an asymptomatic 50-year-old man with a tiny membranous ventricular septal defect. The fan-shaped signal void jet (black arrows) extends from just beneath the aortic valve and ascending aorta (AoA) into the normal-sized right ventricle. The left ventricle (LV) and transverse right pulmonary artery (RP) are normal in size. The long white arrow identifies the right atrial appendage.

left ventricular in character, the heart is labeled double-inlet left ventricle (the most common type); when the morphology is right ventricular in character, then the heart is termed double-inlet right ventricle. If the main ventricular chamber cannot be characterized as either left or right ventricle, then the chamber is referred to as a common ventricle or ventricular chamber. MRI is quite helpful in the evaluation of patients with univentricular hearts and other complex congenital heart lesions. Direct demonstration of right or left ventricular morphology, the relationship between atrioventricular and semilunar valves, and the origins of papillary muscles are all helpful for characterizing the nature of such a ventricle. The interventricular septum in these patients frequently takes an unusual orientation. This and the common association of atrioventricular valvular atresia often necessitate acquisition of coronal as well as off-sagittal sections.

In patients with double-inlet ventricle, both left and right atrioventricular valves empty into a dominant ventricle (Fig. 3-87). Although a rudimentary opposite chamber is usually present, it may only appear as a slit within the posterior or anterior ventricular myocardium. Isolation of the rudimentary (outflow) chamber from atrial inflow is helpful for full characterization of these lesions. In these cases, communication between dominant ventricle and rudimentary ventricular chamber is via a bulboventricular foramen, generally demonstrated in coronal, or even axial section (Fig. 3-88).

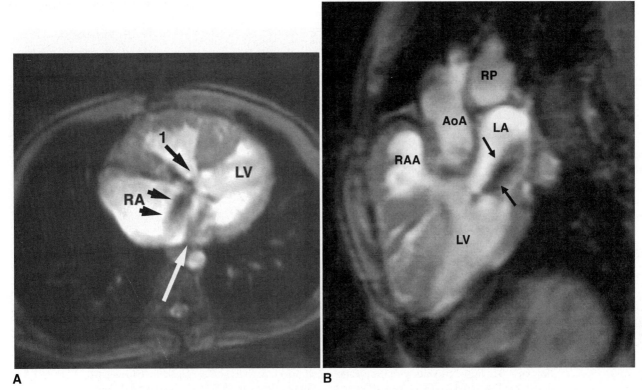

A

B

Figure 3-82   Seven-year-old boy with atrioventricular septal defect. **A.** Axial systolic gradient echo acquisition through the posterior ventricular septal defect (arrow 1). The signal void jet of shunt across the atrioventricular septal defect from the left ventricle (LV) into the dilated right atrium (RA) is shown (short arrows). In addition, a less well visualized shunt (long arrow) across a cleft mitral leaflet into the left atrium is seen. **B.** Oblique sagittal systolic gradient echo acquisition better demonstrates the signal void jet (arrows) from the left ventricle (LV) into the left atrium (LA). The transverse right pulmonary artery (RP) is greater in caliber than the ascending aorta (AoA). RAA, right atrial appendage.

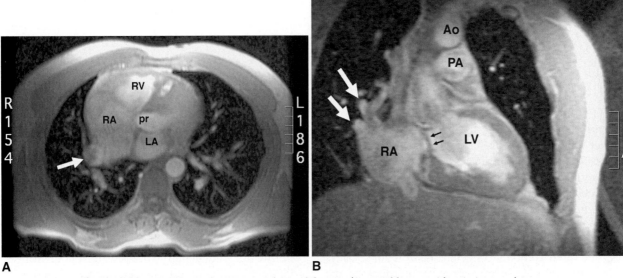

A

B

Figure 3-83   Gradient echo imagery obtained from a 40-year-old man with scimitar syndrome. **A.** Axial diastolic acquisition through the posterior right (pr) aortic sinus of Valsalva. Notice that the heart is rotated into the right chest due to decreased right lung volume. The right ventricle (RV) is normal, and the right atrium (RA) is dilated and confluent with a dilated vascular structure (arrow). A portion of the left atrium (LA) is visualized. **B.** Right anterior oblique sagittal diastolic acquisition through the atrioventricular septum (black arrows). The right pulmonary veins (white arrows) are now seen directly emptying into the right atrium (RA). Notice that the main pulmonary artery (PA) is slightly greater in caliber than the aortic arch (Ao). LV, left ventricle.

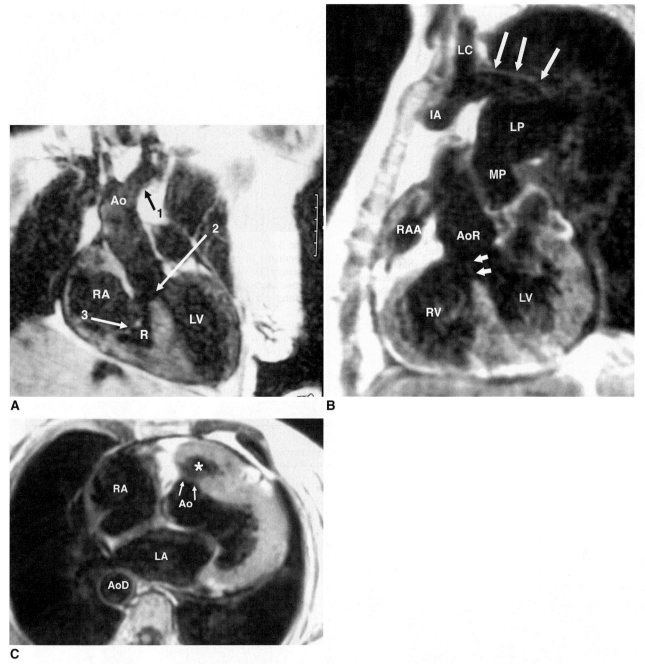

Figure 3-84   Double inversion recovery acquisitions from a 53-year-old woman with tetralogy of Fallot, in whom a Blalock–Taussig shunt was placed as a child. **A.** Off-coronal acquisition. The right-sided aortic arch (Ao) and left-sided innominate artery (arrow 1) are demonstrated. The aortic root lies over the ventricular septal defect (arrow 2), allowing the aorta to have a relationship with both the left ventricle (LV) and the inflow of the right ventricle (R), just distal to the tricuspid valve (arrow 3). RA, right atrium. **B.** Left anterior oblique sagittal acquisition through the aortic root (AoR) and subaortic ventricular septal defect (short arrows). Notice that the right ventricular (RV) myocardium is hypertrophied but is not as thick as the left ventricular (LV) myocardium. The right atrial appendage (RAA) is moderately thickened as well. The left-sided innominate artery (IA) bifurcates to provide the left common carotid artery (LC) and the left subclavian artery (long arrows), which was transected and surgically anastomosed to the left pulmonary artery (LP). Most shunted blood flow is to the left lung; the main pulmonary artery (MP) is smaller than the AoR. **C.** Axial acquisition through the plane of the aortic valve (Ao). The crista supraventricularis (arrows) is displaced anteriorly, causing obstruction of the right ventricular outflow (*) from behind. Notice the hypertrophied right ventricular outflow myocardium. The descending aorta (AoD) in this patient with a right aortic arch is seen to the right of the spine at this level in the chest. The left (LA) and right (RA) atria are normal.

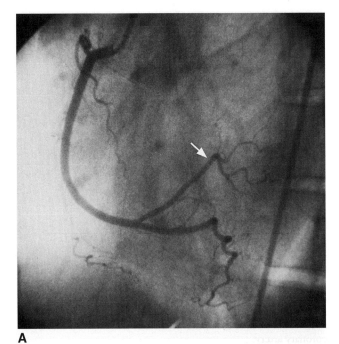

A

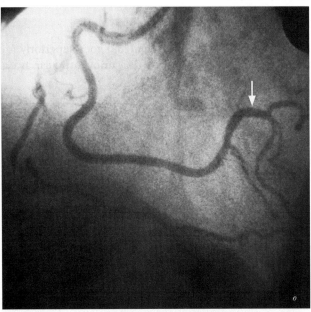

B

Figure 4-11   Two variations of the U-bend (arrow) in the posterior left ventricular branch of the right coronary artery.

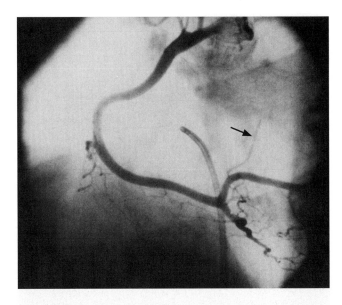

Figure 4-12   Atrioventricular nodal artery. The U-bend of the posterior left ventricular artery is the origin of the atrioventricular nodal artery (arrow) as seen on this LAO view.

Left Circumflex Artery

The left circumflex artery lies in the left atrioventricular groove and may exist only as a vestigial twig or may be so long that it ends by becoming the left posterior descending artery (Figure 4-16). Its major branches are called left circumflex marginal arteries and are numbered first, second, and so on. Because the inferior and left side of the heart is the obtuse border, marginal branches in this location may be called obtuse marginal arteries (Figure 4-17). Late filming of a left coronary artery injection shows the coronary veins. The great cardiac vein, which becomes the coronary sinus, is in the left atrioventricular groove and serves as a landmark for the left circumflex artery.

Left Anterior Descending Artery

The left anterior descending artery lies in the interventricular groove and supplies two distinctive types of branches, septal and epicardial (Figure 4-18). Septal branches go to the interventricular septum, usually along the right ventricular side of the septum, and originate from the left anterior descending artery in a nearly perpendicular direction. The septal branches may themselves have branches, and commonly the first septal branch may have a broomlike appearance. Epicardial branches over the anterolateral wall are called diagonal arteries and number from one to many.

Several characteristics of the left anterior descending artery are unique and help to identify this artery on a

artery and left circumflex arteries originating separately from the left sinus. The left main coronary artery may trifurcate into a left anterior descending artery, an intermediate artery or ramus medianus (Figure 4-14), and the left circumflex artery. The caudal LAO (also called the "spider" view because of the arachnoid shape of the proximal left coronary artery) puts the left main and proximal circumflex arteries in the plane of the film but foreshortens the left anterior descending artery (Figure 4-15).

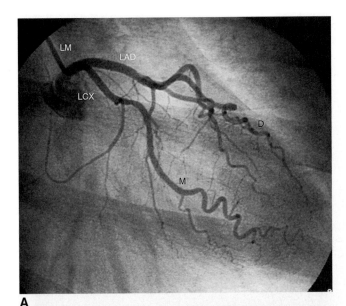

A

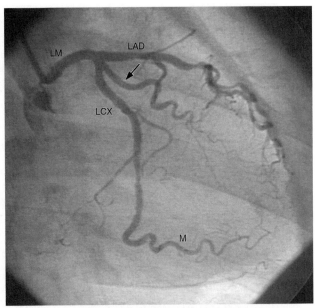

Figure 4-14   Intermediate artery. Intermediate artery (arrow) between the left anterior descending (LAD) and the left circumflex (LCX) arteries. LM, left main artery; M, circumflex marginal branch.

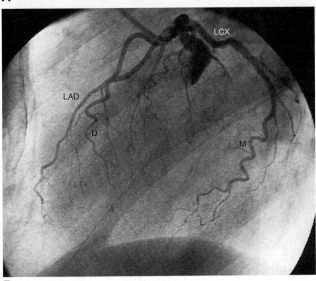

B

Figure 4-13   Left main coronary artery. A, Caudal RAO projection. **B,** Lateral projection. D, diagonal branch; LAD, left anterior descending artery; LCX, left circumflex artery; LM, left main artery; M, circumflex marginal branch.

Cardiac Veins

Identification of the cardiac veins is useful in angiography because they mark the atrioventricular and interventricular boundaries of the chambers. Occasionally they demonstrate anomalies such as persistent left superior vena cava terminating in the coronary sinus, absence of the coronary sinus, or anomalous pulmonary venous connection to the coronary sinus. Veins are distinguished from coronary arteries because the veins opacify several seconds after arterial injection, have less opacification than the corresponding adjacent arteries, are generally larger than the adjacent arteries, and drain into the coronary sinus or a cardiac chamber.

The coronary sinus begins at its opening into the right atrium with its thebesian valve and extends along the left atrioventricular sulcus to the bifurcation with the oblique vein of Marshall. In a normal heart this latter vein is obliterated but when it remains patent it continues as a left superior vena cava. The continuation of the coronary sinus beyond this vein of Marshall is the great cardiac vein. This vein extends beneath the left atrial appendage and becomes the anterior interventricular vein beside the left anterior descending artery.

The left ventricle has veins that lie roughly beside the major arteries (Figure 4-21). The anterior interventricular vein lies adjacent to the left anterior descending artery; it extends superiorly from the apex to pass beneath the left atrial appendage and joins the great cardiac vein beside the left circumflex artery.

coronary angiogram. The anterior descending artery is usually the longest branch of the left coronary artery and ends at the cardiac apex, or occasionally continues to supply most of the inferior septum. The termination characteristically looks like an inverted Y (Figure 4-19). Unlike other branches of the left coronary artery, the left anterior descending artery has numerous septal branches throughout its length (Figure 4-20). A rare septal branch may come from the left main, a diagonal, or a circumflex marginal artery proximally. There is little motion of the left anterior descending artery in contrast to the 1 cm excursion of the left circumflex artery adjacent to the left atrium.

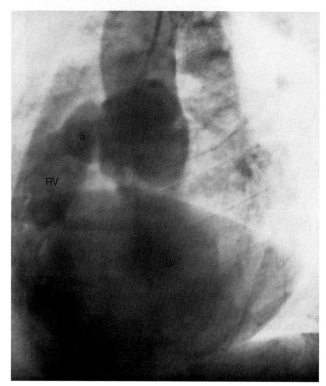

Figure 4-34   Rupture of the right sinus of Valsalva into the right ventricle. An aortic root abscess (a), which caused aortic regurgitation into the left ventricle (LV), later eroded into the right ventricle (RV).

Like the pulmonary valve leaflets, the aortic leaflets are difficult to see during systole, but during diastole they mark the boundary of the left ventricle and the sinuses of Valsalva. The leaflets may occasionally flutter in a person with a high cardiac output or in an elderly patient, possibly related to turbulence immediately beyond the cuspal attachments. During pull-back from the left ventricle to the ascending aorta, subaortic stenosis (fibromuscular dysplasia of the left ventricular outflow tract) can be diagnosed.

ELECTROCARDIOGRAPHY-GATED MULTIDETECTOR ROW COMPUTED TOMOGRAPHY CORONARY ANGIOGRAPHY

Current multidetector row CT (MDCT) has a gantry rotation time of 500 msec or less. Algorithms have been developed to use only data obtained during a portion of the rotation, giving temporal resolution as low as 210 msec in half scan mode or 90 msec in multisector mode. When the data used to reconstruct an image are chosen during slow heart motion in diastole, accurate

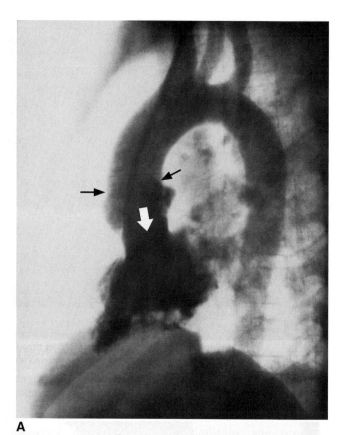

A

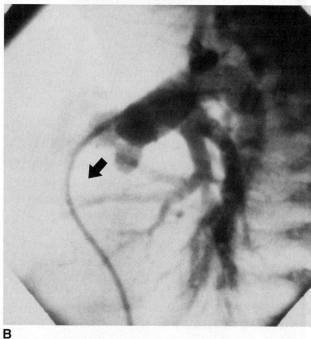

B

Figure 4-35   The tilt of the aortic root. A, Normally a line (large arrow) through the plane of the sinotubular ridge (small arrows) points posteriorly. **B,** In truncus arteriosus, in which both the aorta and the pulmonary arteries originate from the truncal valve, a line (arrow) through the "untucked" valve points anteriorly.

imaging of the coronary arteries can be obtained when gated with an electrocardiogram (ECG). As for MRA, ECG triggering is mandatory for this technique.

For MDCT, the heart rate should be below 65 beats per minute, giving a diastole long enough to image the heart almost without motion. Usually, a bolus test is given in order to target the optimal time to start the acquisition. Usually, about 100 mL of iodinated contrast is delivered through an antecubital vein at a flow rate of 4.0 mL/sec. The breath-hold time, correlated with the scan time, is usually less than 20 seconds. For coronary CT angiography, a retrospective ECG gating technique is applied and images are reconstructed at different R–R intervals.

Numerous studies have been published that compare ECG-gated MDCT with coronary angiography. With 16-detector row CT units, the sensitivity and specificity are around 95% and 93% respectively in the detection of coronary artery stenosis. Noninvasive imaging modalities are still not reaching the level of image quality and temporal resolution of selective coronary angiography and do not allow interventional treatment. Coronary CT angiography still has to find its place in a clinical application. Some potential targets could be to assess normal coronary arteries, to avoid negative invasive angiograms, or in follow-up studies after stent or medical therapies, or to assess bypass graft patency. Figure 4-3 shows a typical result of a normal coronary CT angiography.

INTRAVASCULAR ULTRASOUND

Coronary angiography remains limited by several factors. This technique depicts only the vessel lumen. Angiography does not depict the tissue elements below the intimal surface, and direct visualization of the cross-sectional luminal area is not feasible. Intravascular ultrasound (IVUS) is also very sensitive in detecting plaques (Figure 4-36), as in positive remodeling. This technique also provides accurate qualitative and quantitative data after interventional therapies. IVUS may also provide interesting data about the characterization of plaque (lipid-rich or not). IVUS allows accurate measurement of vessel dimensions when compared to histology and is considered as the gold-standard technique, as angiograms have been shown to be less accurate in dimension measurements.

HEMODYNAMIC STUDIES

During coronary angiography, the operator can easily assess significant (≥75%) and nonsignificant (<50%) stenosis. Nevertheless it is still difficult, in some circumstances, to decide whether a lesion is significant or not,

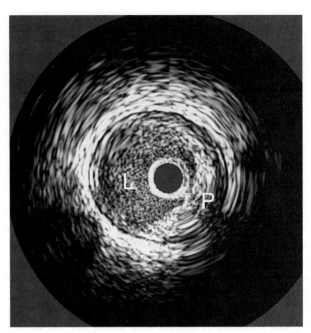

Figure 4-36   Coronary intravascular ultrasound. A coronary plaque (intimal thickening) is depicted from 12 o'clock to 6 o'clock on the right side. Measurement of luminal diameters can be obtained and compared with adjacent IVUS images proximal and distal to the plaque. L, lumen; P, plaque.

especially without noninvasive stress tests or inconclusive results. A technique has been developed to assess the severity of a narrowing by means of hemodynamic measurements. Pressure measurements are obtained simultaneously at the ostium of the coronary artery and beyond the narrowed segment, under pharmacological stress (adenosine). At maximum hyperemia, the ratio of the ostial coronary and distal coronary pressures is obtained. This ratio is called myocardial fractional flow reserve (FFR). The distal coronary artery pressure is obtained with a wire similar in size with the ones used for PTCA. When the FFR is above 0.75, the narrowing is not considered significant and no intervention is performed. The FFR is independent of change in blood pressure and heart rate and also takes account of collateral blood flow to the dependent myocardium. FFR can also easily be performed after angioplasty or stenting, to assess the hemodynamic modification after treatment.

SUGGESTED READING

Amplatz K, Formanek G, Stanger P, Wilson W. Mechanics of selective coronary artery catheterization via femoral approach. *Radiology* 1967;89:1040–1047.

Bech GJ, De Bruyne B, Bonnier HJ, *et al.* Long-term follow-up after deferral of percutaneous transluminal coronary angioplasty of intermediate stenosis on the basis of coronary pressure measurement. *J Am Coll Cardiol* 1998;31:841–847.

CHAPTER 5

Valvular Heart Disease

STEPHEN WILMOT MILLER

Valvular Aortic Stenosis
Chest Film Findings
Imaging Features
Congenital Valvular Aortic Stenosis
Acquired Valvular Aortic Stenosis
Subvalvular Aortic Stenosis
Pathologic Abnormalities
Angiographic Findings
Unusual Subaortic Obstruction
Supravalvular Aortic Stenosis
Classifications
Associated Lesions
Aortic Regurgitation
Chest Film Findings
Angiographic Technique
Magnetic Resonance Imaging Technique
Imaging Findings
Specific Causes of Aortic Regurgitation
Prosthetic Aortic Valves
Mitral Stenosis
Chest Film Findings
Imaging Approach to Mitral Stenosis
Rheumatic Mitral Stenosis
Congenital Abnormalities Causing Left Ventricular Inflow
    Obstruction
Mitral Regurgitation
Chest Film Findings
Angiographic Evaluation
Rheumatic Mitral Regurgitation
Mitral Valve Prolapse
Chordal Rupture
Papillary Muscle Rupture
Papillary Muscle Dysfunction
Imaging Complications of Mitral Valve Replacement
Pulmonary Stenosis and Regurgitation
Chest Film Findings
Valvular Pulmonary Stenosis

Subvalvular Pulmonary Stenosis
Supravalvular Pulmonary Stenosis
Pulmonary Regurgitation
Tricuspid Valve Disease
Tricuspid Stenosis
Tricuspid Regurgitation
Ebstein's Anomaly
Other Imaging Findings

Cardiac imaging in suspected valvular disease determines the involvement of the valves, the extent of the stenosis or regurgitation, and the hemodynamic consequence of the pressure or volume overload on the heart. It also evaluates associated conditions, such as aortic dissection or aneurysm, and ventricular contractility and enlargement.

The chest film serves not only as the initial imaging examination to detect valvular disease but also is the main procedure to visualize any complications such as pulmonary edema and cardiac or aortic dilatation. Imaging the heart chambers with echocardiography, magnetic resonance imaging (MRI), or angiography then follows. Noninvasive Doppler techniques or invasive measurements by catheter allow quantitative hemodynamic evaluations.

Figure 5-1 illustrates the anatomic positions of the heart valves.

VALVULAR AORTIC STENOSIS

A number of features of aortic stenosis at the valvular level are common to several types of pathologic condition; these differ only in the age of the patient and in the degree of severity. The signs include:
- calcification of the leaflets
- thickened leaflets

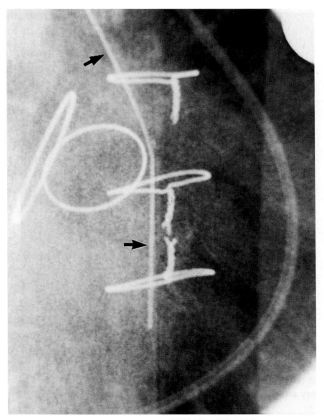

Figure 5-24   Paravalvular leak. A catheter (arrows) has been passed from the aorta beside the Hancock valve into the left ventricle.

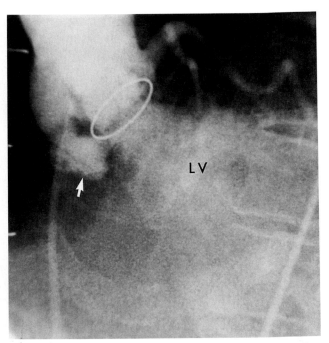

Figure 5-25   Pseudoaneurysm in the aortic root after valve replacement. In the left anterior oblique projection a pseudoaneurysm (arrow) is seen near the anterior aspect of the aortic root; this abscess is in the upper part of the ventricular septum. The left ventricle (LV) is mildly opacified by both valvular and paravalvular regurgitation.

is seen as contrast material beside the sewing ring (Fig. 5-24). The usual cause of late paravalvular regurgitation, and in fact a possibility at any time after valve replacement, is prosthetic endocarditis. When this occurs, the angiographic findings are a fistula between the sinuses of Valsalva and the left ventricle and pseudoaneurysms adjacent to the prosthesis (Fig. 5-25). Vegetations may extend into the valve and cause decreased motion of the leaflets.

MITRAL STENOSIS

Most mitral stenosis is acquired and results from rheumatic carditis that occurred 5–10 years previously. Less common is a left atrial myxoma, thrombus, or a tumor, which may prolapse through the mitral orifice during diastole and create stenosis. Rarely, the calcium in a mitral annulus may be so extensive that the leaflets become thickened and stenotic. Infective endocarditis with a large vegetation and congenital mitral stenosis are unusual causes of an obstructive mitral valve.

Early in the course of rheumatic mitral stenosis in the adult, the pulmonary blood flow redistributes to the upper lobes. Later, the pulmonary arteries enlarge as

pulmonary arterial hypertension develops. Later still, the right ventricle fails, both from a pressure overload from pumping into hypertensive pulmonary arteries and from pulmonary regurgitation from a dilated annulus. In the late stage of rheumatic mitral stenosis, tricuspid regurgitation may develop from the dilated right ventricle or rarely from intrinsic rheumatic disease on the tricuspid valve.

The time course of mitral stenosis in the adult is:
- left atrium enlarges and pulmonary blood flow redistributes to the upper lobes (Fig. 5-26)
- interstitial lung disease with Kerley B lines
- pulmonary arteries enlarge as pulmonary arterial hypertension develops (Fig. 5-27)
- right ventricular enlargement from pressure overload from hypertensive pulmonary arteries
- pulmonary regurgitation from a dilated pulmonary artery
- right ventricular failure
- tricuspid regurgitation (Fig. 5-28).

Box 5-3 summarizes the causes of mitral stenosis.

Chest Film Findings

The chest film in mitral stenosis physiologically reflects the left atrial hypertension. There are signs of left atrial enlargement but the left ventricle is normal in size.

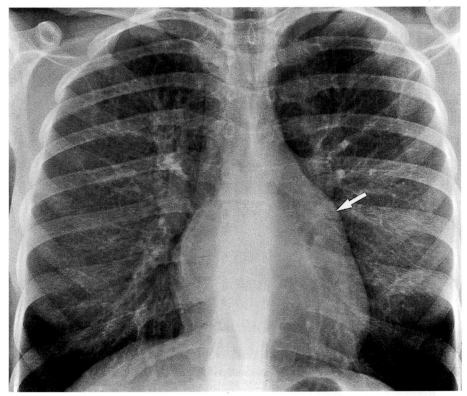

Figure 5-26   Mitral stenosis. The large left atrial appendage (arrow) is rather specific for rheumatic mitral stenosis. The left ventricle has normal size, and the upper lobe vessels are dilated indicating pulmonary venous hypertension.

In the child with a hypoplastic left heart syndrome and congenital mitral stenosis, there is an enlarged heart and pulmonary edema. In the adult with rheumatic heart disease, the onset of mitral thickening and chordal scarring and retraction occurs over such a long period that the lungs have made adaptive changes in the walls of the pulmonary arteries and veins. The lungs have an interstitial pattern that is probably part fibrosis and part edema. Pulmonary edema is visible as an interstitial pattern but not as an acinar pattern, unless there is a complication such as an infected or thrombosed valve. Patients with severe mitral stenosis may rarely have hemoptysis. The site of bleeding is probably in the engorged plexus of vessels around the middle to smaller bronchi. A late sequela of the bleeding is the development of hemosiderosis (Fig. 5-29). These deposits may ossify.

Calcification in the mitral valve is nodular and amorphous. The amount of calcium roughly correlates with the degree of mitral stenosis but, unlike the aortic valve, the mitral valve may be severely stenotic and have no radiologically visible calcification (Fig. 5-30). As a late sequela to the inflammatory carditis in acute rheumatic fever, the left atrium may calcify (Fig. 5-31). These patients have long-standing atrial fibrillation and are at risk for left atrial thrombus and emboli.

Imaging Approach to Mitral Stenosis

You will usually use echocardiography to evaluate abnormalities of the mitral valve. As discussed in Chapter 2, the area of the mitral orifice is measured by ultrasound, and the salient characteristics of mitral stenosis are graded: calcification and mobility in the valve, submitral scarring, and leaflet thickening. Left ventriculography (Fig. 5-32) is needed before percutaneous mitral valvuloplasty to grade mitral regurgitation, as moderate to severe regurgitation precludes the procedure. Occasionally, pulmonary

---

Box 5-3   Causes of Mitral Stenosis

Acquired

Rheumatic (predominant cause)
Prolapse of left atrial tumor or thrombosis
Leaflet deposits from amyloid or carcinoid or
    mucopolysaccharidoses

Congenital

Hypoplastic left heart syndrome
Parachute deformity
Obstructing papillary muscles
Ring of connective tissue on left atrial side of mitral
    annulus

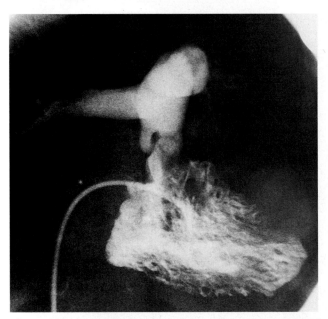

Figure 5-47   Dysplastic pulmonary valve. The sinuses of Valsalva are mildly deformed and eccentric in diastole. The annulus and infundibulum are slightly hypoplastic. The leaflets had little change in systole.

an angiographic appearance that has been likened to 'an open clamshell engulfing the infundibulum' (Fig. 5-48). In addition to the other features of tetralogy of Fallot, the areas of obstruction include the infundibular and supravalvular narrowing. There is usually no poststenotic dilatation of the distal main pulmonary artery.

The annulus of the pulmonary valve may be hypoplastic. The leaflets of the valve and the adjacent main pulmonary artery are usually small and form part of the stenosis (Fig. 5-49).

Congenital absence of the pulmonary valve is usually associated with a ventricular septal defect, annular pulmonary stenosis, and aneurysmal dilatation of the main pulmonary artery and the central part of both the right and left pulmonary arteries. This lesion can occur as an isolated entity but is associated with tetralogy of Fallot. The syndrome may also include a right aortic arch and peripheral pulmonary artery stenoses. The hilar pulmonary arteries may compress the bronchi, leading to hyperinflated lungs.

In Noonan syndrome, many cases have a dysplastic pulmonary valve. Hypertrophic cardiomyopathy

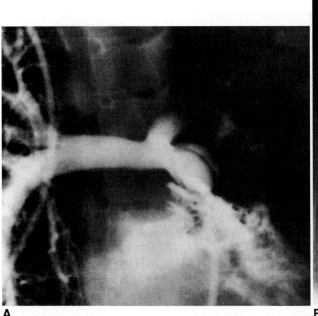

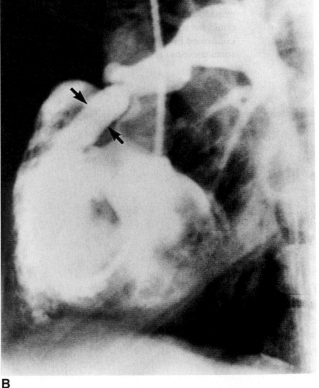

A   **B**

Figure 5-48   Bicuspid pulmonary valve in tetralogy of Fallot. A, The length of the leaflets of the pulmonary valve appears greater than the width of the annulus. In addition to the doming of the leaflets, the infundibulum is hypoplastic. The left pulmonary artery is not seen because of competing flow through a left Blalock–Taussig shunt. **B,** On the lateral view, the hypoplastic infundibulum (arrows) is below the domed pulmonary valve. The left ventricle is opacified through the ventricular septal defect.

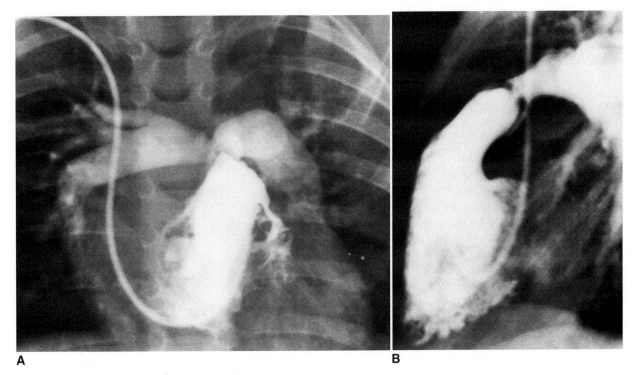

Figure 5-49   Pulmonary valve annulus stenosis. A, The right ventriculogram shows narrowing at the pulmonary valve and supravalvular stenosis involving the bifurcation of the right and left pulmonary arteries. A large trabeculation is seen laterally. **B,** On the lateral view in systole, the leaflets of the stenotic valve are domed and the annulus is small. The main pulmonary artery is mildly hypoplastic.

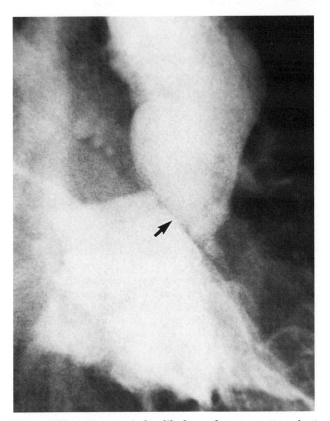

Figure 5-50   Discrete infundibular pulmonary stenosis. A thin membrane is seen as a lucency between the body of the right ventricle and the infundibulum (arrow).

commonly accompanies the pulmonary stenosis as part of the autosomal dominant syndrome.

Subvalvular Pulmonary Stenosis

Subpulmonary obstruction may occur either in the infundibulum or at the junction of the right ventricular body with the infundibulum. Primary infundibular obstruction is a rare malformation which may appear as either a fibrous band or a threadlike cavity through the infundibulum (Fig. 5-50). Discrete narrowing at the level of the crista supraventricularis divides the right ventricle into a main cavity and an infundibular chamber. In this situation, there is contraction of the infundibular chamber during systole, leading to more severe obstruction in addition to its fixed, discrete narrowing. The pulmonary valve may be normal but usually shows slight thickening, presumably because of the turbulence created by the obstruction.

Other types of subpulmonary obstruction result from the muscular hypertrophy of the hypertrophic cardiomyopathies. The right ventricular outflow tract can show dynamic narrowing in idiopathic hypertrophic subaortic stenosis.

Infundibular stenosis frequently coexists with valvular stenosis. This type is not seen until after the patient is several months old, when other signs of right ventricular hypertrophy also become visible. Dynamic infundibular stenosis during systole may appear with a ventricular septal defect. This hypertrophy in the outflow tract decreases the left-to-right flow across the ventricular septal defect (Gasul phenomenon) and may cause stenosis that increases with age (Fig. 5-51).

Hypoplasia of the crista supraventricularis is the main element in the infundibular stenosis in tetralogy of Fallot. The underdevelopment of the infundibulum is associated with displacement of the crista above the ventricular septal defect. About half of patients with tetralogy of Fallot also have valvular pulmonary stenosis, in which case the pulmonary annulus is also small.

Obstructing muscular bands of the right ventricle, an abnormality that has also been called double-chambered right ventricle, may cause an obstruction either in the body of the right ventricle or higher in the infundibular region. These muscle bundles are seen as filling defects in the right ventricle, which may not contract. When the anomalous muscle occurs in the true right ventricular cavity, its location is variable; it may extend from the apex as a triangular mass on the posteroanterior projection or from the tricuspid valve to the junction of the infundibulum as a diagonal or wedge-shaped filling defect (Fig. 5-52).

Supravalvular Pulmonary Stenosis

In supravalvular pulmonary stenosis, the pulmonary arteries are hypoplastic and may have segmental focal stenoses. In tetralogy of Fallot, there frequently is mild focal stenosis at the origin of the left and occasionally of the right main pulmonary artery. Occasionally the left pulmonary artery is absent. Rare causes of supravalvular pulmonary stenosis include Williams syndrome, carcinoid syndrome from an abdominal tumor with liver metastases, extrinsic stenoses from mediastinal fibrosis or tumor, and rubella.

These stenoses have a wide spectrum of morphologic appearance, from a short, discrete area of narrowing to long, diffuse hypoplastic segments involving several branches. There may be poststenotic dilatation with variable caliber of the peripheral artery. When evaluating the central variety of pulmonary stenosis at cardiac catheterization, you should use cranial angulation of the beam for the right ventriculogram so that the bifurcation of the main pulmonary artery into the right and left arteries is completely visible. Gay and colleagues have classified the stenoses for surgical therapy according to their location. Type 1 has a single stenosis in the main pulmonary artery. Type 2 occurs at the bifurcation of the main with the right and left pulmonary arteries. Type 3 has only peripheral or branch stenoses. Type 4 is a mixture of the other types (Fig. 5-53).

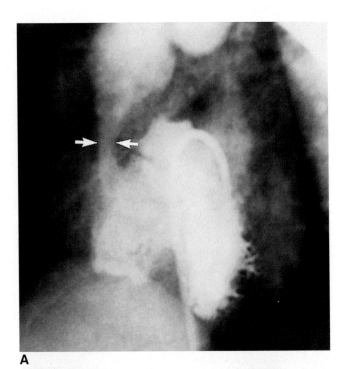

A

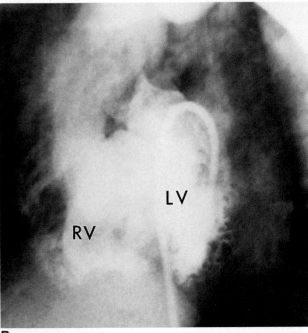

B

Figure 5-51   Gasul phenomenon. The catheter has crossed the patent foramen ovale to enter the left ventricle (LV). In this lateral projection the body of the right ventricle (RV) has become opacified through the ventricular septal defect. In systole (**A**), the infundibulum (arrows) is markedly narrow, while in diastole (**B**), no subvalvular stenosis exists.

Diffuse pulmonary artery hypoplasia is a congenital malformation that may occur in isolation or with cardiac anomalies (Fig. 5-54). Centrally located segmental stenoses may be congenital (Fig. 5-55), while peripheral pulmonary arterial stenosis usually are secondary to

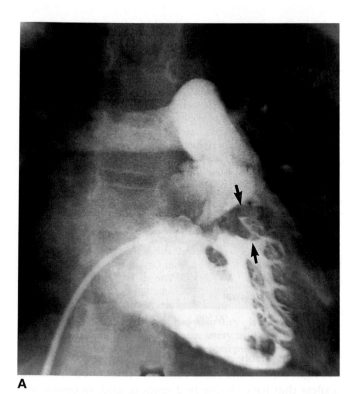

A

B

Figure 5-52   Double-chambered right ventricle. A, A muscular bar (arrows) extends horizontally from near the tricuspid annulus to the anteroseptal wall and separates the body and infundibular sections of the right ventricle. **B,** A second type of obstructing muscular band (arrows) runs vertically on the free wall of the right ventricle and angles across the bottom of the infundibulum.

other diseases (Fig. 5-56). Scarred lung from previous pneumonia, bullous emphysema, recanalized pulmonary emboli, and pulmonary arteritis from Takayasu's disease are common causes.

Acquired supravalvular pulmonary stenosis in the form of pulmonary banding is created intentionally to reduce torrential pulmonary blood flow. The band is correctly positioned above the pulmonary annulus in the main pulmonary artery but may migrate distally causing unwanted branch stenosis (Fig. 5-57). A band placed too close to the pulmonary valve may cause leaflet thickening.

Pulmonary Regurgitation

Pulmonary regurgitation usually is acquired and results from pulmonary arterial hypertension. A congenital cause of pulmonary regurgitation is absence of the pulmonary valve, which is associated with tetralogy of Fallot. This malformation has large pulmonary arteries and a narrow pulmonary annulus creating a stenosis. Conversely, if a patient known to have tetralogy of Fallot paradoxically has large pulmonary arteries, he or she also has pulmonary regurgitation and an absent pulmonary valve.

The general rule that structures on each side of a regurgitant valve dilate is valid in chronic severe pulmonary regurgitation. The right ventricle and the central pulmonary arteries become large.

TRICUSPID VALVE DISEASE

Tricuspid Stenosis

The chest film in tricuspid valve disease is quite variable. The abnormalities in tricuspid stenosis follow the principle that the chamber behind a severe stenosis is large. Although right atrial enlargement is always seen, the right ventricle and the left heart frequently are also big because tricuspid stenosis is a late sequela of rheumatic mitral stenosis. The superior vena cava and azygos vein are enlarged. In congenital Ebstein's anomaly, the film may be strikingly specific with its right atrial and right ventricular enlargement. The right atrium at the junction with the superior vena cava has an unusual rounded appearance (Fig. 5-58). In other types of tricuspid valve disease, the plain film shows nonspecific cardiac enlargement, occasionally with dilatation of the superior and inferior vena cava. In rheumatic heart disease, the features of mitral stenosis predominate: left atrial enlargement and pulmonary artery enlargement. Tricuspid valve calcification rarely may be seen at fluoroscopy. Tricuspid annular calcification has the same causes as mitral annular calcification, namely, dystrophic degeneration from aging and from chronic severe right ventricular hypertension (Fig. 5-59).

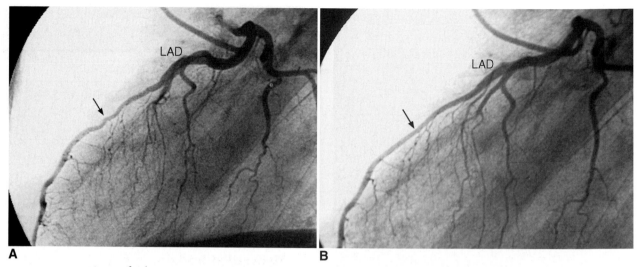

Figure 6-24   Intramyocardial bridge. The mid left anterior descending artery (LAD; arrow) is narrowed and deformed during systole (**A**), as it courses into the myocardium, but has a normal caliber at end diastole (**B**).

Because the bridge is usually eccentric, you should obtain views in at least two orthogonal projections.

The septal arteries, which are also intramural, normally show no change in size between systole and diastole. Septal arteries from the left anterior descending artery may occlude during systole in diseases that increase left ventricular wall tension such as aortic stenosis, hypertensive heart disease, and idiopathic hypertrophic subaortic stenosis.

Coronary Dissection

The angiographic appearance of dissection is a linear or spiral lucency within the arterial lumen, which represents the intimal flap (Figure 6-25). The dissection may occlude the distal artery or, as in the aorta, have a false channel with stasis of the contrast medium. Spontaneous dissection occurs in the coronary arteries as it does in most medium-sized arteries (Figure 6-26). It is seen in

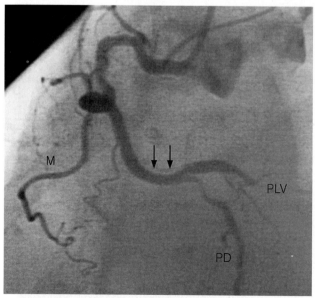

Figure 6-25   Coronary artery dissection. Spontaneous dissection of the distal right coronary artery (arrows), starting just prior to the posterior descending artery (PD), with the membrane of the dissection extending into posterior left ventricular branches (PLV). M, marginal branch.

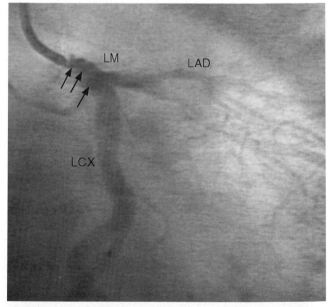

Figure 6-26   Aortic dissection. Patient with type A aortic dissection and ischemic signs on admission electrocardiogram. The aortic dissection involved also the ostium (arrow) of the left main coronary artery (LM) and impaired the coronary blood flow, especially in the left anterior descending artery (LAD).

pregnancy, Marfan syndrome, and chest trauma. Coronary dissection may occur secondary to an aortic dissection with a retrograde tear. The angiographic catheter may lift a plaque and initiate the downstream tear. After transluminal angioplasty, a short dissection cleft is frequently seen but rarely extends beyond the length of the balloon.

CONGENITAL ANOMALIES OF THE CORONARY ARTERIES

Coronary anomalies can be defined morphologically or hemodynamically. Morphologic variations can arise in the origin, course, or termination of the coronary arteries. These variations may be isolated anomalies or be related to certain forms of congenital heart disease. Coronary anomalies may cause cardiac ischemia. In this group are four major anomalies:

- coronary fistulas
- origin of the left coronary artery from the pulmonary artery
- congenital coronary artery stenosis or atresia
- origin of the left coronary artery from the right sinus of Valsalva with the left main coronary artery passing between the right ventricular infundibulum and the aorta.

The morphologic classification is used in this discussion.

Anomalies of Origin

Although the usual origin of the left and right coronary arteries is the left and right sinuses of Valsalva respectively, ectopic coronary arteries can arise above the sinuses in the ascending aorta, within the posterior (noncoronary) sinus, low within the sinus adjacent to the leaflet, within the commissure, or in a subvalvular location. The conus artery frequently originates as a separate ostium in the right sinus of Valsalva. There may be no left main artery if the left anterior descending and circumflex arteries arise separately from the left sinus of Valsalva. A common anomaly is the left circumflex artery arising from the right sinus of Valsalva and passing behind the aorta into the left atrioventricular groove (Figure 6-27). When the left coronary artery originates from the right sinus of Valsalva, it may

- pass anterior to the right ventricular outflow tract
- go between the pulmonary artery and the aorta (Figure 6-28), or
- circle posteriorly behind the aorta to get to the left ventricle.

Similarly, when the right coronary artery originates from the left sinus of Valsalva by passing between the aorta and the right ventricular infundibulum, it forms an acute angle at its ostium and may be compressed by the two great vessels. If the anomalous right coronary, originating

from the left sinus of Valsalva, courses anteriorly to the aorta, it should not produce any symptom, unless it is diseased (Figure 6-29). Rarely a left coronary artery arises from the right sinus of Valsalva, assumes an intramyocardial course by traversing through the crista supraventricularis, then continues as the left anterior descending and circumflex arteries in their usual locations.

The coronary arteries may have ectopic origins from structures other than the aorta. In this situation, the anomalies include:

- origin of the left coronary artery from the pulmonary artery
- origin of the right coronary artery from the pulmonary artery
- origin of both coronary arteries from the pulmonary artery
- origin of the conus artery from the pulmonary artery with branching to both right and left circumflex arteries
- origin of the left circumflex artery from the pulmonary artery.

The most common of these is the left coronary origin from the pulmonary artery. This entity, the Bland–White–Garland syndrome, is seen in infants who have a myocardial infarction in the first few months of life. Coronary arteriography shows an empty left sinus of Valsalva. The right coronary artery supplies collaterals to the left coronary artery, which fills in a retrograde direction to opacify the pulmonary arteries (Figure 6-30). The infantile left ventricle may have a segmental wall motion abnormality like that seen in coronary disease in the adult. Left ventricular aneurysms and mitral regurgitation can produce congestive heart failure. Left ventricular aneurysms may completely regress after corrective coronary surgery.

Anomalies of Origin and Course

Major coronary anomalies of location are those that go behind the aorta, between the aorta and the pulmonary artery, or anterior to the right ventricular infundibulum. A prime example of this group is the isolated single coronary artery, which can originate from either the left or right sinus of Valsalva (Figure 6-31). The most common anomaly is origin of the left circumflex artery from the right coronary artery with a course that goes behind the aorta before supplying the usual circumflex territory. You can usually see this retroaortic course on a right anterior oblique left ventriculogram and it will alert you to the anomaly. Other common variations include the left anterior descending artery coming from the conus artery, and the posterior descending artery continuing around the apex as a long left anterior descending artery (Figure 6-32).

The anomaly that can cause an angina and sudden death is the aberrant coronary artery that goes between

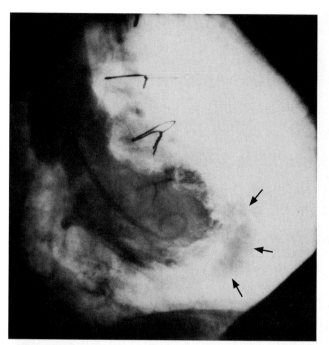

Figure 6-48 False left ventricular aneurysm after ventriculotomy. The extraluminal collection of contrast (arrows) at the apex occurred at the site of a puncture to vent air as the patient came off coronary bypass. The blood is constrained by the adjacent pericardium and mediastinal scarring.

false aneurysms resulting from myocardial infarct are on the posterolateral and diaphragmatic sides of the left ventricle (Figure 6-49).

The left ventriculogram demonstrates a discrete saccular aneurysm whose neck is considerably smaller than the internal circumference of the saccule. Contrast material may not flow into the false aneurysm until late in systole, and it may oscillate into and out of the neck of the aneurysm without exiting from the left ventricle. Because of the narrow communication with the left ventricular chamber, the opacification of the false aneurysm may persist for many seconds after the injection has ended (Figure 6-50). Frequently the false aneurysm is bigger than the left ventricle and, in fact, may enlarge over serial examinations. This has prognostic significance in that false aneurysms have a high propensity to rupture. Rupture of a true aneurysm is rare, occurring in less than 4% of several necropsy series. In contrast, postmortem series indicate that approximately 45% of false aneurysms rupture. Echocardiography is also the first modality of choice when a false aneurysm is suspected.

The coronary arteries in patients with false aneurysms are also severely diseased. However, reflecting the posterior and diaphragmatic location of most false aneurysms, there is frequent occlusion of the right coronary artery, whereas, with true aneurysm, occlusion is more common in the left coronary artery.

Cardiac false aneurysm (or changes that look like aneurysms) may result from diseases other than coronary artery disease. Congenital diverticula of the left ventricle may be confused with false aneurysm but they usually are smaller and occur at the apex. The African cardiomyopathies that have apical aneurysms usually can be distinguished by both their clinical course and the absence of coronary disease. The rare submitral aneurysms found in black Africans are not caused by ischemia. These aneurysms have a narrow neck originating between the mitral annulus and the posteromedial papillary muscle. The large sac lies beneath the left atrium and displaces it superiorly.

RUPTURE OF THE INTERVENTRICULAR SEPTUM

Clinical Presentation

Rupture of the interventricular septum is an uncommon complication of myocardial infarction that occurs in about 1% of those who sustain infarction. If not surgically treated, more than 90% of those with rupture die within 1 year. The appearance of a new systolic murmur within hours to weeks after myocardial infarction, particularly if associated with biventricular failure or cardiogenic shock, suggests ventricular septal defect or ruptured papillary muscle.

Common abnormalities in chest radiographs of patients with a ruptured septum are signs of interstitial or alveolar pulmonary edema and left ventricular enlargement (Table 6-2). Enlargement of other chambers is inconstant. Almost half will show pleural effusions, enlargement of the pulmonary arteries, and signs of pulmonary venous hypertension. Occasionally, an unusual configuration of the heart will suggest the presence of an aneurysm in addition to the septal rupture (Figure 6-51).

Left Ventricular Signs

Doppler echocardiography is a good noninvasive technique to demonstrate ventricular septal rupture. During left ventriculography, almost all patients have at least one segment with akinesis or dyskinesis. The posterolateral wall is hyperkinetic in some patients, suggesting that the exaggerated motion is partly compensating for the other segments of the ventricle. The septum is always akinetic or dyskinetic.

In the right anterior oblique view, you will see opacification of the pulmonary artery during left ventriculography. This view superimposes the two ventricles. The most inferior wall visible is the diaphragmatic wall of the right ventricle. If the left ventricular diaphragmatic wall is akinetic, the adjacent right ventricular wall behaves similarly. In the left anterior oblique projection, contrast

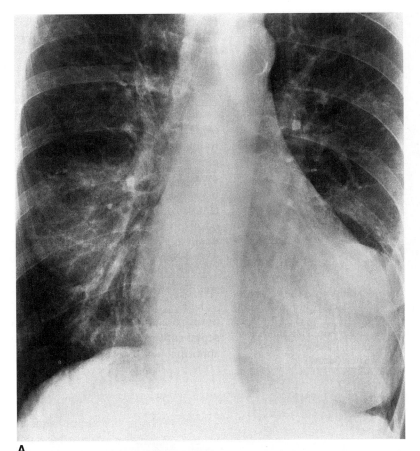

A

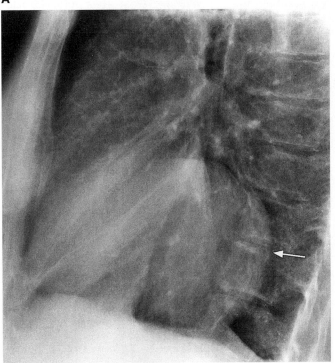

B

Figure 6-49   Contour abnormality in left ventricular false aneurysm. The patient had a false aneurysm develop at the site of a true aneurysm. **A,** The anterolateral and apical location is typical of a true aneurysm. **B,** The lateral chest film shows an aneurysm in the posterolateral wall (arrow), more typical of a false aneurysm. The chest film cannot distinguish between the types of aneurysm but is more useful for diagnosing their presence and whether they have increased in size.

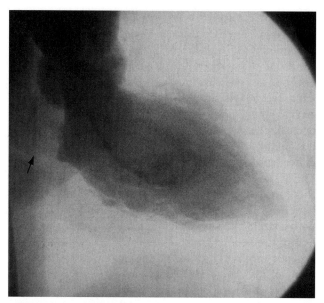

Figure 6-53   Papillary muscle dysfunction. Mitral regurgitation (arrow) has resulted from akinesis of the inferior wall after an infarct.

and its adjacent left ventricular free wall. For example, hypokinesis, akinesis, or aneurysm may produce any degree of mitral regurgitation (Figure 6-53).

Complete rupture of a necrotic papillary muscle is quite rare and, because of its acute severity, usually causes the death of the patient. Recent surgical advances have made survival possible for some individuals if this lesion is recognized early. The more frequent clinical event is rupture of only one head of the papillary muscle, allowing the attached chordae to partially support both mitral leaflets and to limit somewhat the amount of regurgitation.

Ventriculographic Signs

The left ventriculographic signs of papillary muscle dysfunction include left ventricular enlargement, an akinetic wall that contains a papillary muscle or an adjacent left ventricular aneurysm, calcification in a papillary muscle, and any degree of mitral regurgitation. The papillary muscle may be quite large, swollen with edema associated with myocardial infarction. In the setting of free mitral regurgitation after myocardial infarction, one or both heads of a papillary muscle must have ruptured, indicating the need for emergent mitral valve replacement. Echocardiography should be performed immediately following acute myocardial infarction if mitral valve regurgitation is suspected.

SUGGESTED READING

ACC/AHA guidelines for percutaneous coronary intervention (revision of the 1993 PTCA guidelines). *J Am Coll Cardiol* 2001;37:2215-2238.

Ambrose JA, Winters SL, Arora RR, *et al.* Angiographic evolution of coronary artery morphology in unstable angina. *J Am Coll Cardiol* 1986;7:472-478.

Ambrose JA. Plaque disruption and the acute coronary syndromes of unstable angina and myocardial infarction: if the substrate is similar, why is the clinical presentation different? *J Am Coll Cardiol* 1992;19:1653-1658.

Baim DS, Kline H, Silverman JF. Bilateral coronary artery-pulmonary artery fistulas. Report of five cases and review of the literature. *Circulation* 1982;65:810-815.

Bogaty P, Brecker SJ, White SE, *et al.* Comparison of coronary angiographic findings in acute and chronic first presentation of ischemic heart disease. *Circulation* 1993;87:1938-1946.

Bolli R. Myocardial "stunning" in man. *Circulation* 1992;86: 1671-1691.

Brown BG, Gallery CA, Badger RS, *et al.* Incomplete lysis of thrombus in the moderate underlying atherosclerotic lesion during intracoronary infusion of streptokinase for acute myocardial infarction: quantitative angiographic observations. *Circulation* 1986;73:653-661.

Brown BG, Zhao ZQ, Sacco DE, *et al.* Lipid lowering and plaque regression. New insights into prevention of plaque disruption and clinical events in coronary disease. *Circulation* 1993;87:1781-1791.

Cabins HS, Roberts WC. Left ventricular aneurysm, intra-aneurysmal thrombus and systemic embolus in coronary heart disease. *Chest* 1980;77:586-590.

Cabins HS, Roberts WC. True left ventricular aneurysm and healed myocardial infarction. Clinical and necropsy observations including quantification of degrees of coronary arterial narrowing. *Am J Cardiol* 1980;46:754-763.

Davies MJ. A macro and micro view of coronary vascular insult in ischemic heart disease. *Circulation* 1990;82(Suppl. 2):II-38-II-46.

Davies SW, Marchant B, Lyons JP, *et al.* Coronary lesion morphology in acute myocardial infarction: demonstration of early remodeling after streptokinase treatment. *J Am Coll Cardiol* 1990;16:1079-1086.

Faxon DP, Ryan TJ, Davis KB, *et al.* Prognostic significance of angiographically documented left ventricular aneurysm from the coronary artery surgery study (CASS). *Am J Cardiol* 1982; 50:157-164.

Feldman RL, Nichols WW, Pepine CJ, *et al.* Hemodynamic significance of the length of a coronary arterial narrowing. *Am J Cardiol* 1978;41:865-871.

Fellows KE, Freed MD, Keane JF, *et al.* Results of routine preoperative coronary angiography in tetralogy of Fallot. *Circulation* 1975;51:561-566.

Formanek A, Nath P, Zollikoffer C, *et al.* Selective coronary arteriography in children. *Circulation* 1980;61:84-95.

Fuster VF, Badimon L, Badimon JJ, *et al.* The pathogenesis of coronary artery disease and the acute coronary syndromes. *N Engl J Med* 1992;326:242-250, 310-318.

Gould KL, Kirkeeide RL, Buchi M. Coronary flow reserve as a physiologic measure of stenosis severity. *J Am Coll Cardiol* 1990;15:459-474.

Gould KL, Kirkeeide RL. Assessment of stenosis severity. In: Reiber JHC, Serruys PW, eds. *State of the art in quantitative coronary arteriography*. Dordrecht: Martinus Nijhoff, 1986:209.

Greenberg MA, Fish BG, Spindola-Franco H. Congenital anomalies of the coronary arteries: classification and significance. *Radiol Clin North Am* 1989;27:1127-1146.

Harding MB, Leither ME, Mark DB, et al. Ergonovine maleate testing during cardiac catheterization: a 10 year perspective in 3,447 patients without significant coronary artery disease or Prinzmetal's variant angina. *J Am Coll Cardiol* 1992;20:107-111.

Higgins CB, Lipton MJ. Radiography of acute myocardial infarction. *Radiol Clin North Am* 1980;18:359-368.

Irvin RG. The angiographic prevalence of myocardial bridging in man. *Chest* 1982;81:198-202.

Jacoby DS, Mohler ER III, Rader DJ. Noninvasive atherosclerotic imaging for predicting cardiovascular events and assessing therapeutic interventions. *Curr Atheroscler Rep* 2004;6:20-26.

Kahn K, Fisher MR. MRI of cardiac pseudoaneurysm and other complications of myocardial infarction. *Magn Reson Imaging* 1991;9:159-164.

Kaski JC, Rosano GMC, Collins P, et al. Cardiac syndrome X. Clinical characteristics and left ventricular function. *J Am Coll Cardiol* 1995;25:807-814.

Kereiakes DJ, Topol EJ, George BS, et al. Myocardial infarction with minimal coronary atherosclerosis in the era of thrombolytic reperfusion. *J Am Coll Cardiol* 1991;17:304-312.

Kimbiris JB, Iskandrian AS, Segal BL, et al. Anomalous aortic origin of coronary arteries. *Circulation* 1978;58:606-615.

Kloner RA, Przyklenk K, Patel B. Altered myocardial states: the stunned and hibernating myocardium. *Am J Med* 1986;80 (Suppl. 1A):14.

Lee J, Choe YH, Kim HJ, et al. Magnetic resonance imaging demonstration of anomalous origin of the right coronary artery from the left coronary sinus associated with acute myocardial infarction. *J Comput Assist Tomogr* 2003;27:289-291.

Levin DC, Gardiner GA Jr. Complex and simple coronary artery stenoses: a new way to interpret coronary angiograms based on morphologic features of lesions. *Radiology* 1987;164:675-680.

Liberthson RR, Dinsmore RE, Bharatic S, et al. Aberrant coronary artery origin from the aorta. Diagnosis and clinical significance. *Circulation* 1974;50:774-779.

Liberthson RR, Sagar K, Berkoben JP, et al. Congenital coronary arteriovenous fistula. Report of 13 patients, review of the literature and delineation of management. *Circulation* 1979;59:849-854.

Manning WJ, Li W, Edelman RR. A preliminary report comparing magnetic resonance coronary angiography with conventional angiography. *N Engl J Med* 1993;328:828-832.

Marcus ML, Schelbert HR, Skorton DJ, et al. *Cardiac imaging: a companion to Braunwald's heart disease*. Philadelphia, PA: WB Saunders, 1991.

Massie BM, Botvinick EH, Brundage BH, et al. Relationship of regional myocardial perfusion to segmental wall motion. A physiologic basis for understanding the presence and reversibility of asynergy. *Circulation* 1978;58:1154-1163.

Megnien JKL, Sene V, Jeannin S, et al. Coronary calcification and its relation to extracoronary atherosclerosis in asymptomatic hypercholesterolemic men. *Circulation* 1992;85:1799-1807.

Meizlish JL, Berger HJ, Plankey M, et al. Functional left ventricular aneurysm formation after acute anterior transmural myocardial infarction. *N Engl J Med* 1984;311:1001-1006.

Miller SW, Boucher CA. Assessing the adequacy of myocardial perfusion in man: anatomic and functional techniques. *Radiol Clin North Am* 1985;23:589-596.

Miller SW, Dinsmore RE, Greene RE, et al. Coronary, ventricular, and pulmonary abnormalities associated with rupture of the interventricular septum complicating myocardial infarction. *AJR* 1978;131:571-577.

Mizuno K, Horiuchi K, Matui H, et al. Role of coronary collateral vessels during transient coronary occlusion during angioplasty assessed by hemodynamic, electrocardiographic and metabolic changes. *J Am Coll Cardiol* 1988;12:624-628.

Morbidity from coronary heart disease in the United States, NHLBI Data Fact Sheet. Bethesda, MD: National Heart, Lung, and Blood Institute, 1990.

Motoyasu M, Sakuma H, Ichikawa Y, et al. Prediction of regional functional recovery after acute myocardial infarction with low dose dobutamine stress cine MR imaging and contrast enhanced MR imaging. *J Cardiovasc Magn Reson* 2003;5:563-574.

Nassir K, Budoff MJ, Post WS, et al. Electron beam CT versus helical CT scans for assessing coronary calcification: current utility and future directions. *Am Heart J* 2003;146:969-977.

Neufeld HN, Schneeweiss A, eds. *Coronary artery disease in infants and children*. Philadelphia, PA: Lea & Febiger, 1983.

Petersen SE, Voigtlander T, Kreitner KF, et al. Late improvement of regional wall motion after the subacute phase of myocardial infarction treated by acute PTCA in a 6-month follow-up. *J Cardiovasc Magn Reson* 2003;5:487-495.

Pierard LA, Albert A, Henrard L, et al. Incidence and significance of pericardial effusion in acute myocardial infarction as determined by two-dimensional echocardiography. *J Am Coll Cardiol* 1986;8:517-520.

Pijls NHJ, de Bruyne B, Bech JW, et al. Coronary pressure measurement to assess the hemodynamic significance of serial stenoses within one coronary artery. *Circulation* 2000;102:2371-2377.

Pijls NHJ, de Bruyne B, Peels K, et al. Measurement of fractional flow reserve to assess the functional severity of coronary artery stenoses. *N Engl J Med* 1996;334:1703-1708.

Proudfit WL, Shirey EK, Sheldon WC, et al. Certain clinical characteristics correlated with extent of obstructive lesions demonstrated by selective cine-coronary arteriography. *Circulation* 1968;38:947-954.

Reddy K, Gupta M, Hamby RI. Multiple coronary arteriosystemic fistulas. *Am J Cardiol* 1974;33:304-306.

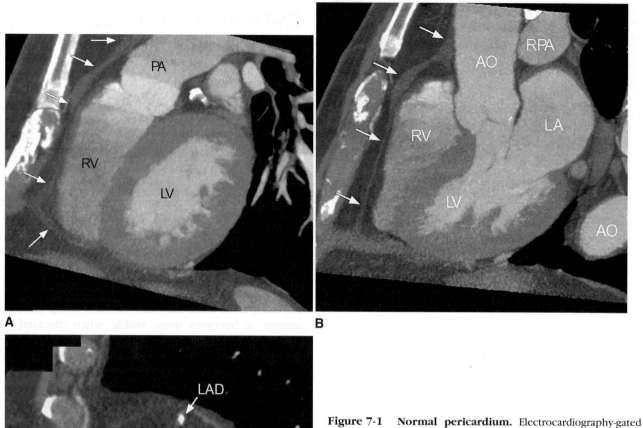

Figure 7-1   Normal pericardium. Electrocardiography-gated CT appearance of normal pericardium in sagittal reconstruction (**A**) and oblique aortic root long axis reconstruction (**B**) show the pericardium (arrows) extending 3 cm upwards on the pulmonary artery (PA) and aorta (AO), where the pericardial reflection site is located. **C**, Ventricular short-axis reconstruction shows pericardium separating epicardial fat (*) from pericardial fat. Note left anterior descending coronary artery (LAD) running in the epicardial fat. LA, left atrium; LV, left ventricle, RPA, right pulmonary artery; RV, right ventricle.

Normal Appearance on Chest Imaging

The visceral and parietal pericardium and the fluid in the pericardial space cannot usually be differentiated on computed tomography (CT) or magnetic resonance imaging (MRI) because the thickness of the pericardial layers is below the limits of the resolution. If a 'thickened pericardium' is described, it usually refers to the combination of visceral pericardium, pericardial fluid, and parietal pericardium. On CT, secondary signs are helpful to differentiate the cause of the thickening of the pericardial complex. Nodularity and enhancement of the thickened pericardium is suggestive of metastatic disease. Calcification indicates chronic pericarditis.

A smoothly thickened pericardial contour is suggestive of, however not diagnostic of, pericardial effusion. One great aid in imaging the pericardium is the fat that covers the outside of the parietal pericardium (pericardial fat) and the fat over the surface of the heart (epicardial fat). On CT and MR, the normal thickness of the pericardium between the sternum and the right ventricular free wall is about 2–3 mm.

Laterally, the pericardium is usually not visible on CT. On MRI images, chemical shift artifacts may cause the pericardium to look like a thick black line in the frequency encoding direction. Special techniques can be used to investigate the different components of the pericardial contour: Phase contrast images allow for detection of

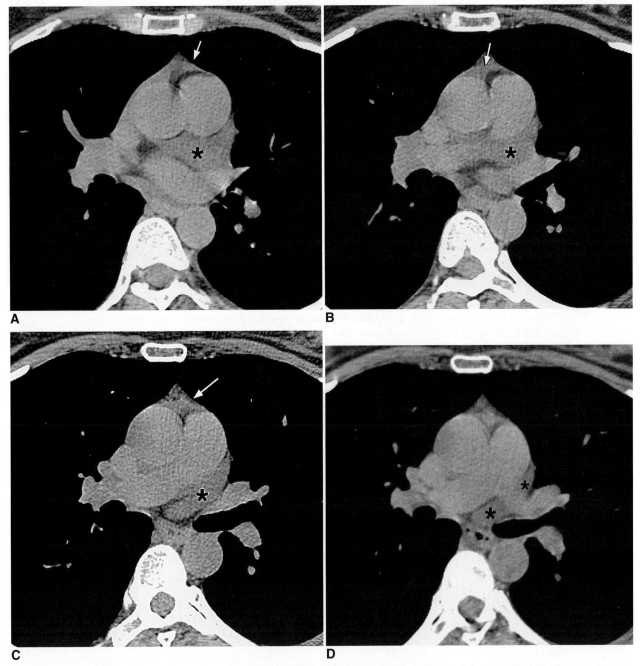

Figure 7-2   Superior recess. Electrocardiography-gated CT slices from calcium scoring show superior recessus (*) posterior to main pulmonary artery and wrapping around left pulmonary artery. Note the superior extent of the pericardial space anterior to the aorta and pulmonary artery (arrows).

freely moving fluid within the pericardial space. Gradient echo images also are bright where fluid is in motion.

Pericardial Effusion

The normal pericardial space in the adult can be distended with 150–250 mL of fluid acutely before cardiac tamponade results. Cardiac tamponade is caused by excess fluid in the pericardial space, which compresses the heart and thus causes a low cardiac output state. In tamponade, the cardiac size on the chest radiograph is slightly to markedly increased. The heart may have a water-bottle appearance in which both sides are rounded and displaced laterally (Figure 7-4). The differential diagnostic considerations for a water-bottle heart are global cardiomegaly, large anterior mediastinal mass, or pericardial effusion. If you are lucky, you may see the Oreo® cookie sign on the lateral chest x-ray (Figure 7-5).

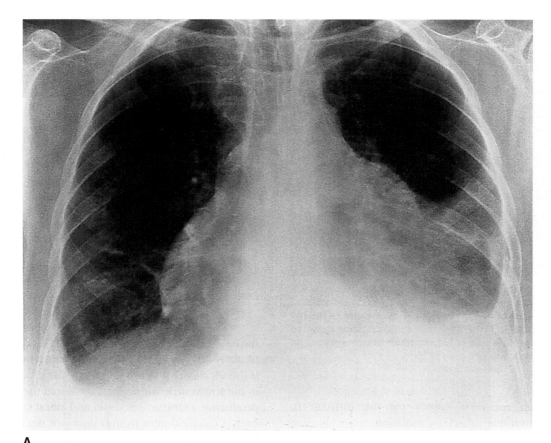

A

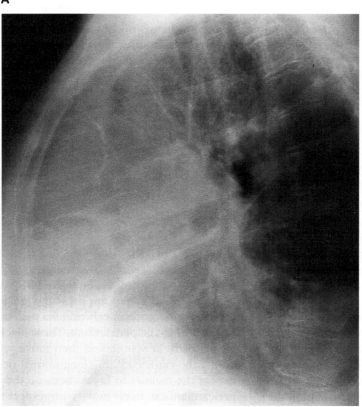

B

Figure 7-9   Dressler syndrome. A, A large, pericardial effusion and bilateral pleural effusions developed 6 weeks after myocardial infarct. Note the unusual rounding of the pericardium over the left atrial appendage. **B,** The lateral film shows a dense anterior mediastinum, reflecting the tense upward bowing of the pericardium. (With permission from Miller SW. Imaging pericardial disease. *Radiol Clin North Am* 1989;27:1113–1125.)

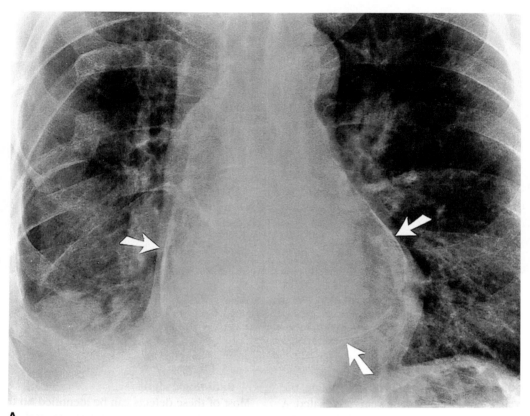

A

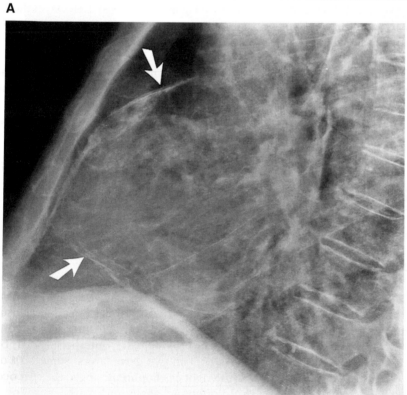

B

Figure 7-10   Constrictive pericarditis with eggshell calcification. 'Eggshell calcification' outlines the heart border (arrows) over both ventricles and the right atrium.

Cardiac Lesions in AIDS

Myocarditis is a common autopsy finding in patients who have died from AIDS, with nearly half having disease in the heart or pericardium. Even though these patients have multiple infections, an agent is rarely identified in the heart. The histopathologic picture is a focal lymphocytic myocarditis. Many infectious agents are occasionally cultured, such as *Mycobacterium avium-intracellulare, Toxoplasma* (Figure 7-30), *Cryptococcus,* Cytomegalovirus, and human immunodeficiency virus (HIV). Kaposi's sarcoma, which is histologically difficult to distinguish from angiosarcoma, and lymphoma are the major pericardial and heart tumors (Figure 7-31). The pericardium frequently has fibrinous pericarditis from uremia or infection and may have a moderate effusion. Vegetations of both infective and nonbacterial endocarditis have been found on all four heart valves. Congestive heart failure with pulmonary edema from left ventricular failure may have a similar clinical presentation as a dilated cardiomyopathy. The right ventricle may be dilated from pulmonary artery hypertension secondary to pulmonary infection or emboli.

Cardiomyopathies

Cardiomyopathies are heart muscle diseases in which congenital, pericardial, valvular, and coronary causes have been excluded by appropriate clinical, hemodynamic, or imaging methods. Primary cardiomyopathies have an unknown etiology whereas secondary cardiomyopathies have an etiologic diagnosis and therefore are potentially reversible with appropriate therapy. Alcoholic, Adriamycin (doxorubicin), and ischemic cardiomyopathies are examples of known causes and produce similar clinical signs, such as ventricular failure, but may require different therapy.

Classification

The WHO/ISFC Task Force classifies primary cardiomyopathies as:
- dilated cardiomyopathy
- hypertrophic cardiomyopathy
- restrictive cardiomyopathy
- arrhythmogenic right ventricular cardiomyopathy/dysplasia (ARVC/ARVD)
- unclassified cardiomyopathies.

Box 7-3   Cardiac Thrombus by Location

LEFT ATRIUM

Mitral valve disease
Atrial fibrillation
Tumor from pulmonary veins

RIGHT ATRIUM

Embolic
    Thromboembolism
    Tumor
        Renal cell carcinoma
        Hepatocellular carcinoma
Foreign body

LEFT VENTRICLE

Cardiomyopathy
Myocardial infarction with scar or aneurysm
Vegetation from endocarditis on mitral valve

RIGHT VENTRICLE

Trauma
Cardiomyopathy
Myocardial infarction with scar or aneurysm
Vegetation from endocarditis on tricuspid valve

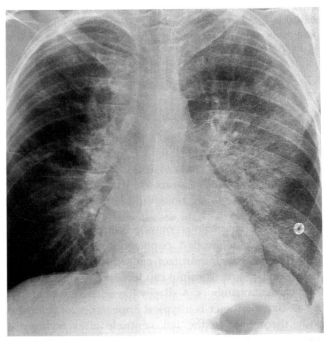

Figure 7-30 *Toxoplasma* **myocarditis in a patient with AIDS.** Although the heart size is normal, 200 mL of pericardial fluid was present at autopsy. Bronchopneumonia is seen in both lungs.

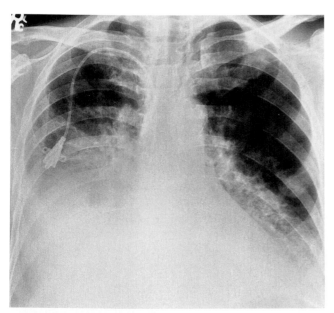

Figure 7-31 Lymphocytic myocarditis. Lymphocytic myocarditis in the immunodeficiency syndrome appearing like a dilated cardiomyopathy. Large, bilateral pleural effusions partially mask a dilated heart with a small pericardial effusion.

Although many patients fit easily into one of these groups, many have features that overlap several categories.

Dilated Cardiomyopathy

Dilated cardiomyopathy causes dilatation of both right and left ventricles. Typically the left ventricle is enlarged with global hypokinesis, whereas the right ventricle is less dilated and typically has a less severe contraction abnormality. Mild mitral and tricuspid regurgitation are common because of the ventricular dilatation. Patients with this condition have decreased ejection fractions with reduced stroke volumes and may have decreased cardiac output. Systolic function is depressed, but diastolic function is nearly normal. As the left ventricle dilates to a moderate degree, segmental wall motion abnormalities may appear. For example, the apex may be akinetic. Mural thrombi are frequently found in the apex and have a laminated appearance.

Because globally decreased wall motion is not unique to this abnormality, cardiac imaging not only measures the left ventricular ejection fraction but also helps exclude other types of heart disease. The chest film generally shows cardiomegaly and pulmonary venous hypertension with little or no pulmonary edema (Figure 7-32). The paradox of a huge heart and clear lungs is a diagnostic clue that a dilated cardiomyopathy may be present. Global reduction in left ventricular wall motion may also be seen in acute viral myocarditis; in eosinophilic myocarditis; and as atypical presentation of other types of cardiomyopathies such as those with infective etiologies (Chagas disease), granulomatous heart disease (sarcoid), and infiltrative heart disease (amyloid) (Figure 7-33). Peripartum cardiomyopathy (Figure 7-34) also has global hypokinesis of both ventricles and occurs during the last trimester of pregnancy or during the first several months post partum.

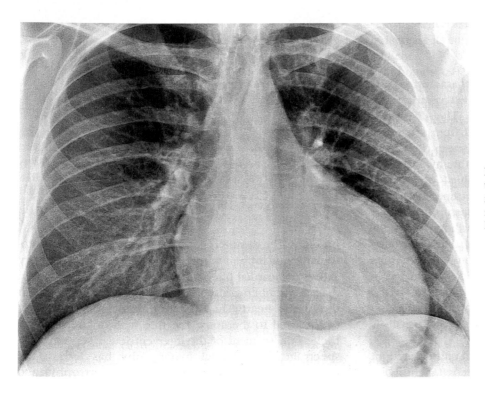

Figure 7-32 Dilated cardiomyopathy. The heart shows enlargement of all four chambers. The azygous vein and superior vena cava are slightly dilated, reflecting high central venous pressure.

side as the thoracic and abdominal viscera do. In situs solitus, the right atrium is on the right side of the mediastinum and the left atrium is on the left side. In situs inversus, the morphologic right atrium is on the left side and the left atrium lies on the right side. In situs ambiguus, right and left sides cannot be determined because the lungs and abdomen are symmetric. For example, in asplenia there are two right (trilobed) lungs and both atria are morphologically right atria. In polysplenia there are two (bilobed) left lungs and both atria are morphologic left atria.

In most people, the major portion of the heart lies slightly to the left of midline. The cardiac apex denotes the location of the heart within the thorax. Dextrocardia (Fig. 8-2), levocardia (Fig. 8-3), and mesocardia then indicate the possible positions of the heart. Using this terminology, a *cardiac malposition* is any heart that does not have a leftward cardiac axis in situs solitus. A malposition includes dextrocardia in situs solitus and levocardia in situs inversus (Fig. 8-4), as well as dextrocardia in situs inversus. All these positions represent deviation from normal embryologic development without necessarily implying any hemodynamic or morphologic derangement.

In primary dextrocardia, the main defect is in the heart. There are two types of *primary dextrocardia*: (1) dextroversion, where the heart is rotated or pivoted so that its apex lies on the right side with the atria as a fulcrum; and (2) mirror-image dextrocardia. In *secondary dextrocardia*, the heart is normal but the mediastinum is shifted to the right because of extracardiac abnormalities that involve the lungs, pleura, or skeleton (Box 8-1). Examples of the

---

Box 8-1　Types of Dextrocardia

Primary Dextrocardia

Dextroversion: The left ventricle is to the left of the right ventricle, as it is in the normal heart
Mirror-image Dextrocardia: The left ventricle is to the right of the right ventricle

Secondary Dextrocardia

Skeletal causes
- Scoliosis
- Sternal or rib deformity

Lung causes
- Pneumonectomy
- Collapse
- Pneumothorax
- Unilateral airtrapping

Pleural causes
- Diaphragmatic hernia with displacement of the gut into left thorax.

---

latter include pneumothorax, congenital herniation of the gastrointestinal tract into the thorax, and thoracolumbar scoliosis (Fig. 8-5).

Atrial Morphology

With rare exceptions, the morphology of the atria corresponds closely with the situs of the tracheobronchial tree

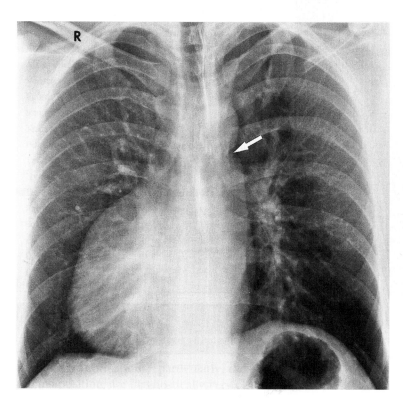

Figure 8-2　Dextrocardia. The cardiac apex lies on the right side, while the abdominal and tracheobronchial structures are on their normal sides. Slight rib notching and an indentation in the descending aortic shadow (arrow) denote coarctation of the aorta. A ventricular septal defect is reflected in the large pulmonary arteries.

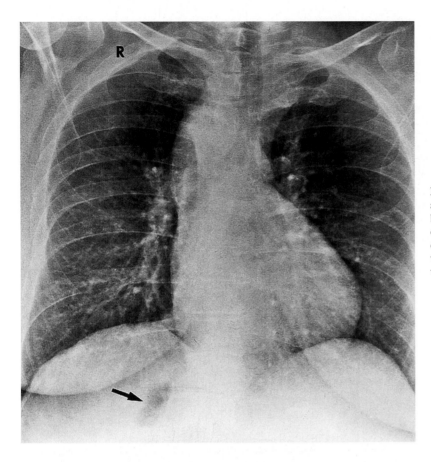

Figure 8-3   Levocardia. The right-sided stomach bubble (arrow) and the asymmetric main stem bronchi with the left-sided epiarterial bronchus are diagnostic of situs inversus. Therefore, the left cardiac apex, which represents levocardia, is discordant with the body situs. Tetralogy of Fallot is present with a right aortic arch.

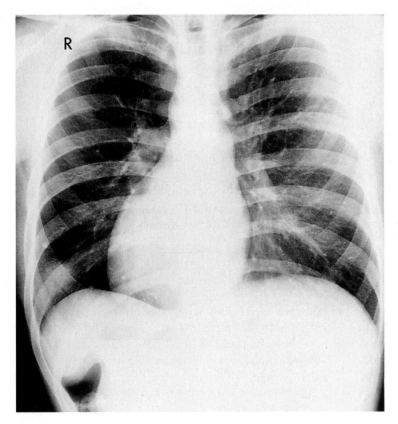

Figure 8-4   Situs inversus. The right and left sides of the abdomen and thorax are reversed in a mirror-image fashion. The spleen, stomach bubble, and lowest leaf of the diaphragm are on the right side of the abdomen. The left-sided lung has an epiarterial bronchus, indicating a morphologic right lung.

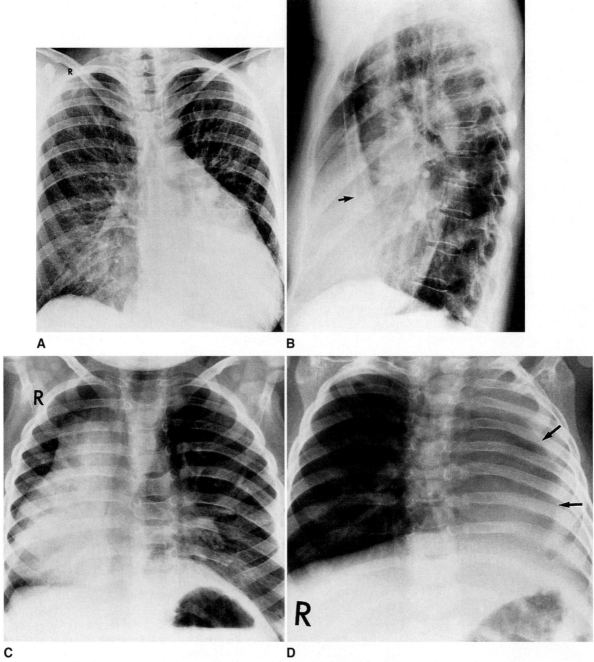

Figure 8-5   Secondary dextrocardia caused by positional changes of the heart and mediastinum. A, B, Levoposition caused by severe pectus excavatum (arrow). **C,** Hypoplasia of the right lung producing dextroposition. **D,** Agenesis of the left lung. The arrows show the extent to which the right lung has herniated across the anterior mediastinum to lie in the left hemithorax. Normal ventricles.

and the abdominal viscera. Of the various criteria for distinguishing between right and left atria, the most reliable are the shape of the atrial appendage and the connection to the inferior vena cava (Table 8-1). The right atrial appendage is broad and pyramidal, while the left atrial appendage is thin with a narrow neck. The inferior vena cava almost always connects with the right atrium. This is

true even in the 'absence' of the inferior vena cava and azygos continuation. In this entity, there is no intrahepatic portion of the cava but the hepatic veins connect to the subdiaphragmatic portion of the inferior vena cava, which joins the right atrium.

The superior vena cava is a poor landmark of atrial morphology because bilateral cavae may be present or the

Table 8-1   Normal Atria

Right Atrium	Left Atrium
Broad appendage	Thin appendage
Inferior vena cava connection	Pulmonary vein connection
Coronary sinus	
Valves of the inferior vena cava (eustachian)	
Valve of the coronary sinus (thebesian)	
Fossa ovalis	
Crista terminalis	

right superior vena cava may be absent, and there may be a connection of either the right or left superior vena cava into either atrium or into the coronary sinus. As an example, in situs inversus totalis, the morphologic right atrium is on the left side and the morphologic left atrium lies on the right side of the body, while the right-sided lung has two lobes and the left-sided lung has three lobes. When thoracic isomerism exists in the heterotaxy syndrome, bilateral morphologic right atria are seen in the asplenia syndrome and bilateral left atria in polysplenia.

Ventricular Morphology

When the right and left ventricles are normal, identification of the two ventricles is relatively simple (Table 8-2). The normal right ventricle has coarse, trabeculated walls when compared with the smooth-walled left ventricle. The right ventricle has a contractile muscle called the conus or infundibulum between the tricuspid and pulmonary valves, while the left ventricle has mitral–aortic continuity with no intervening muscle. The right ventricle has trabeculations and papillary muscles on its septum,

Table 8-2   Normal Ventricles

Right ventricle	Left ventricle
Coarse, trabeculated walls	Smooth walls
Contractile muscle (conus, infundibulum between tricuspid and pulmonary valves	Mitral aortic continuity with no intervening muscle
Trabeculation and papillary muscles on septum	Septum free from trabeculations and papillary muscles
Tricuspid atrioventricular valve	Bicuspid (mitral) atrioventricular valve
Complex triangular shape	Spheroidal shape

whereas in the left ventricle these structures are not present on the septum. A bicuspid (mitral) atrioventricular valve is a part of the left ventricle, while a tricuspid atrioventricular valve is part of the right ventricle, although either of these valves may have a cleft or be absent.

When some of the structures used to identify the ventricles are congenitally absent or malformed, the identification of the two ventricles becomes confusing. To clarify this situation, identify the three anatomic segments in the normal ventricle:
- the inlet or inflow tract
- the trabecular part
- the outlet or outflow tract.

The inlet segment in the right ventricle is smooth and adjacent to the tricuspid valve; in the left ventricle it is between the papillary muscles and the mitral valve. The trabecular segment constitutes the body of the ventricle distal to the insertion of the papillary muscles. This trabeculated segment is a key feature in the distinction between the two ventricles. In the right ventricle, there are large, coarse trabeculations, prominent in both systole and diastole. In the left ventricle, the wall is smooth in diastole but has fine trabeculations during systole. The ventricular outlet portion of the right ventricle is a tubular muscular structure, the conus, which separates the inlet and outlet valves. In the left ventricle, the outlet is smooth and has no muscle between the inlet and outlet valves.

When one or more of these three ventricular segments is absent, the heart may be called a single ventricle. Similar terminology for hearts that lack at least one of the three ventricular segments are:
- single ventricle
- univentricular heart
- common ventricle
- double-inlet left ventricle
- double-inlet right ventricle
- undifferentiated ventricle.

There is general agreement that an inflow tract must be present for a chamber to be considered a ventricle. The trabecular portion determines whether the chamber is of the right or left ventricular type. In these instances, the single ventricle consists of one large chamber that receives both atrioventricular valves. (Note that this definition excludes mitral or tricuspid atresia.) If only the trabecular and outflow segments are present, this structure is called an outlet chamber. Examples of such hearts are the univentricular heart of the left ventricular type, with or without a rudimentary outflow chamber.

Difficulties arise in this classification scheme when part of an inlet or outlet valve overrides the septum. In this situation, rather than make an arbitrary decision, a description of the amount of overriding is appropriate. In general, when either the inlet or outlet valve is associated with more than 50% of a ventricle, it is considered to be a part of that ventricle. Examples of this condition

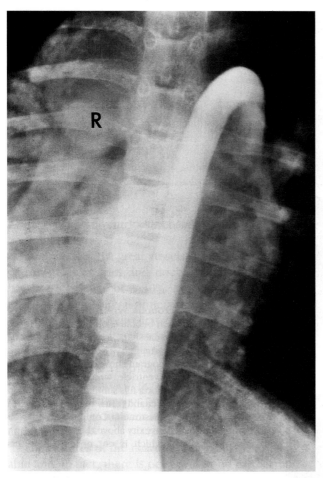

Figure 8-14 Hemiazygos continuation in a patient with polysplenia and dextrocardia. An injection into the left femoral vein opacified the hemiazygos vein adjacent to the costovertebral sulcus before it emptied into a left superior vena cava.

of the great arteries. Atrioventricular discordance with concordance of the ventricles and great arteries, a rare malformation, is called ventricular inversion.

Congenitally Corrected Transposition of the Great Vessels (Levotransposition of the Great Arteries)

In 1875 Rokitansky reported a form of transposition in which blood passed in normal serial fashion through the pulmonary and systemic circuits. The right atrium was connected to the left ventricle, which was connected to the pulmonary artery. On the oxygenated side of the lungs, the left atrium was connected to the right ventricle, which was connected to the aorta. The atrioventricular valves always correspond with their ventricles, even when there is atrioventricular discordance. That is, the mitral valve is a left ventricular structure, and the tricuspid valve is a right ventricular structure. In congenitally corrected transposition of the great vessels, the aorta lies to the left of and anterior to the pulmonary artery, while the pulmonary valve lies to the right and posterior. The aortic

valve is usually somewhat anterior to the pulmonary valve, although the two great vessels may be exactly lateral to each other. The ascending aorta frequently has an unusual course, passing in a direction toward the left shoulder so that occasionally a distinctive contour in the left side of the mediastinum is visible on the chest film.

If there are no other defects, this malformation causes no hemodynamic problems and may go undetected during a normal life span. Unfortunately, associated malformations are the rule, and their site and severity determine the clinical course. Ventricular septal defects are frequent (Fig. 8-15) and may be large enough to cause pulmonary arterial hypertension. These defects are usually in the membranous septum adjacent to the pulmonary valve; muscular defects and supracristal defects are less common. Generally, the left-sided atrioventricular valve (i.e., the valve between the left atrium and the right ventricle) is displaced slightly into the ventricle in a manner resembling Ebstein's anomaly. If the displacement is more than a few millimeters (because the tricuspid valve is usually displaced to the apex by that amount), the diagnosis of Ebstein's anomaly is quite likely. Pulmonary stenosis is frequently associated with ventricular septal defect and may be caused by a malformed valve, a subpulmonary membrane, aneurysms of the membranous ventricular septum, or, rarely, accessory tissue in the atrioventricular valve or a muscular bar in the subpulmonary region.

Angiography begins with the conventional postero-anterior and lateral projections. These establish the atrioventricular connections, the morphology of the ventricles, and the position of the aorta and pulmonary artery. As you discover associated malformations, you will frequently need additional injections in specialized views, particularly in cases of dextrocardia. The position of the venous and arterial catheters frequently give the first clue to a corrected transposition (Fig. 8-16). In situs solitus and levocardia, the venous catheter passes through the heart in the midline to reach the pulmonary arteries. On the lateral view, the catheter in the pulmonary artery is posterior to its usual location, which is where the aorta should be in normal hearts. The retrograde arterial catheter has a distinctive curve in the ascending aorta as its course becomes convex medially and to the left before entering the heart. On the lateral view, the aortic catheter is anterior and superior to the venous catheter. The venous and arterial catheters indicate the fundamental relationship between the aorta and the pulmonary artery in corrected transposition with situs solitus and levocardia; the pulmonary artery lies to the right and posterior, while the aorta is anterior and to the left.

In corrected transposition with situs solitus and levocardia, angiography initially consists of right and left ventriculography in the posteroanterior and lateral projections. In the posteroanterior projection, the ventricles lie nearly side by side with the interventricular septum,

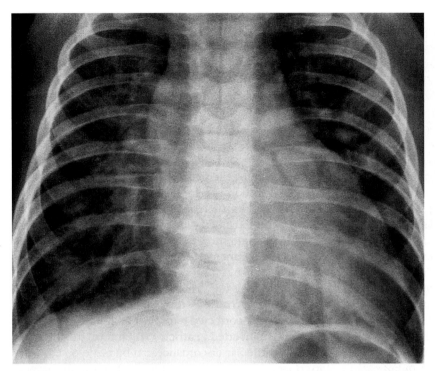

Figure 8-15   Congenitally corrected transposition of the great arteries with ventricular septal defect. The leftward course of the ascending aorta is not apparent on the chest film. The leftward cardiac apex represents the right ventricle, which is enlarged because of the ventricular septal defect. The main pulmonary artery is not part of the mediastinal interface with the lung because it is central; the hilar and peripheral pulmonary arteries are large from the left-to-right shunt.

seen on end. The left ventricle lies slightly inferior to the right ventricle and has a triangular shape, with the mitral valve lying medially and to the right. The mitral valve of the left ventricle connects to the right atrium and lies in continuity with the pulmonary valve. The left ventricular outflow region is short and vertically oriented, with the anterior leaflet of the mitral valve on the medial side and the membranous portion of the interventricular septum forming the superior and lateral wall.

In the lateral view, the left ventricle appears to 'stand on its apex' with a conical shape whose apex is in the diaphragmatic–sternal angle. The anterior wall of the left

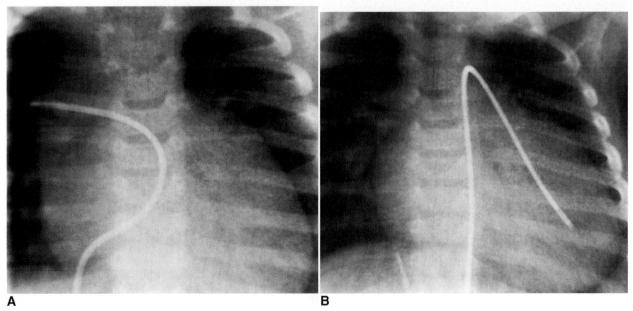

A   B

Figure 8-16   Catheter positions in congenitally corrected transposition of the great arteries. A, The catheter in the inferior vena cava passes through the right atrium and left ventricle to end in the pulmonary artery. **B,** The retrograde aortic catheter ends in the right ventricle. The ascending aorta lies to the left of the pulmonary valve.

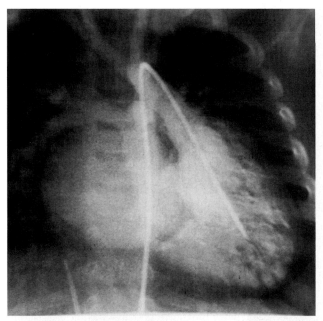

Figure 8-19   Ebstein's anomaly in congenitally corrected transposition of the great arteries. Injection into the right ventricle has resulted in severe regurgitation into the left atrium. In contrast to isolated Ebstein's anomaly, the tricuspid leaflets are poorly seen, and have little apical displacement. A ventricular septal defect has allowed opacification of the pulmonary arteries.

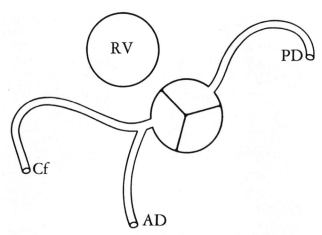

Figure 8-20   Coronary arteries in corrected transposition of the great arteries. The aortic valve is anterior and to the left of the right ventricular infundibulum (RV). The posterior descending artery (PD) originates posteriorly and follows the atrioventricular groove between the left atrium and right ventricle. The circumflex artery (Cf) lies in the atrioventricular groove between the right atrium and left ventricle, while the anterior descending artery (AD) follows the interventricular sulcus. With situs solitus, the coronary arteries appear to be the mirror image of those in the normal heart.

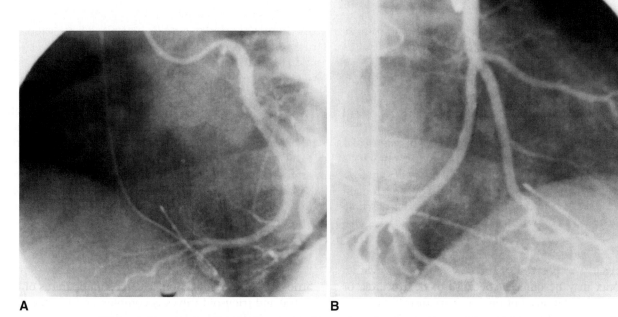

A   **B**

Figure 8-21   Situs solitus and congenitally corrected transposition of the great arteries. The right coronary artery is inverted from its location in the normal heart in the left (**A**) and right (**B**) anterior oblique projections.

Peripherally, the chordae or the papillary attachments may cross the septal defect to attach in the contralateral ventricle. Most of these valves represent a type of complete atrioventricular canal defect. An overriding atrioventricular valve has its annulus on both sides of a septal defect. An atrioventricular valve then may be straddling, overriding, or both.

Ventriculoarterial Discordance

The next stage in the segmental analysis concerns the connections and relations of the great arteries with respect to the ventricles. There are a number of ventriculoarterial malformations, most of which are a transposition of the great arteries or one of its variants. A complete description of a ventriculoarterial defect involves three aspects:

- the anteroposterior relationship of the aorta and pulmonary artery
- the connection of the aorta and the pulmonary artery to the right and left ventricles
- the presence of a conus beneath the aortic and pulmonary valves.

If a conus is present, there is contractile tissue between the atrioventricular and semilunar valves.

The most common variety of ventriculoarterial discordance is transposition of the great arteries. In this sense, 'transposition' means that the two great arteries are abnormally placed with respect to the interventricular septum: the aorta connects to the right ventricle and the pulmonary artery to the left ventricle. As an illustration, complete dextrotransposition of the great arteries exists when the aorta is anterior and to the right and connected to the right ventricle, while the pulmonary artery is posterior and to the left and connected to the left ventricle. The term partial transposition applies to variations that do not meet the strict criteria of complete transposition, and includes double-outlet right ventricle and double-outlet left ventricle.

Complete Dextrotransposition of the Great Arteries

In 1797 Baillie described the heart of an infant in which the aorta connected to the right ventricle and the pulmonary artery to the left ventricle. The term 'transposition of the aorta and pulmonary artery' is ascribed to Farre in 1814. Since that time there has been controversy about whether it should be defined by the abnormal anteroposterior position of the great arteries or by the abnormal connections to the ventricles. Transposition of the great arteries is a ventriculoarterial abnormality in which the aorta originates above the right ventricle and the pulmonary artery originates over the left ventricle.

After tetralogy of Fallot, complete transposition of the great arteries is the second most common cause of cyanosis from heart disease in infancy. In this malformation, the systemic and pulmonary circulations connect in parallel, in contrast to the serial connection in the normal infant. The blood flow through the lungs returns to the left atrium and to the left ventricle only to pass again through the lungs; in a similar fashion, the systemic venous and arterial circulations form a closed loop. For life to be sustained, mixing must occur between these two circuits. Therefore, one of the objectives of imaging is to determine the location and amount of these intracardiac or extracardiac shunts. The foramen ovale is almost always patent but is too small for adequate mixing. Occasionally, a secundum atrial septal defect will allow a large shunt to provide adequate mixing of oxygenated blood at this level.

Ventricular septal defects occur in about one-third of babies with transposition and, when present, may result in congestive heart failure from the large blood flow. Extracardiac shunts may occur, as in patent ductus arteriosus or with bronchopulmonary connections to the pulmonary vascular bed. The ductus arteriosus remains patent in one-fourth to one-half of infants who do not receive prostaglandin E1 and allows blood to flow from the pulmonary artery to the aorta if the pulmonary vascular resistance is high, and from the aorta to the pulmonary artery when the high fetal pulmonary artery pressures fall below the systemic blood pressure.

Besides the ventricular septal defect, the other major associated malformation is obstruction to blood entering the pulmonary arteries. About one-fourth of those with transposition of the great arteries have some form of pulmonary stenosis. The site of obstruction is usually in the subpulmonary region and it has a variety of causes:

- anomalous attachment of the mitral valve
- accessory endocardial tissue
- subpulmonary membrane
- subpulmonary fibromuscular tunnel
- aneurysm of the membranous outflow tract.

Valvular pulmonary stenosis also occurs from a unicuspid or bicuspid valve. Dynamic pulmonary stenosis is common in those patients with an intact ventricular septum and is caused by systolic anterior motion of the mitral valves, like that in idiopathic hypertrophic subaortic stenosis.

The typical chest radiograph in the first few days of life of a child with transposition of the great arteries shows mild cardiomegaly, a narrow superior mediastinum, and increased size of the pulmonary vessels that is consistent with a left-to-right shunt. All these signs are variable and, in fact, the chest radiograph may appear normal. The size of the pulmonary vessels depends on the amount of blood carried by them: if the degree of mixing between the pulmonary and systemic circuits is small or if there is some type of pulmonary stenosis, the pulmonary vessels will be small; if there are large intracardiac or extracardiac shunts, the pulmonary vessels are large (Fig. 8-22).

ventricular septal defect in relation to the aorta and pulmonary artery. In the more common type, the ventricular septal defect is adjacent to the aorta with the pulmonary outflow situated on the far side of the right ventricle. In the less common type, the Taussig–Bing heart, the ventricular septal defect is adjacent to the pulmonary outflow, while the aorta arises on the far side of the right ventricle. The aorta is usually to the right of the pulmonary artery, either slightly to the front or directly to the side, but it may arise in front of the pulmonary artery. Although there are rare exceptions, bilateral conus is a major criterion for distinguishing double-outlet right ventricle from tetralogy of Fallot or complete transposition of the great arteries. Bilateral conus is recognizable by muscle between each atrioventricular valve and the semilunar valves. These features place the aortic and pulmonary valves on approximately the same level in the transverse plane.

In addition to the ventriculoarterial malformation and the requisite ventricular septal defect, there are usually a large number of associated anomalies. Subpulmonary stenosis is frequent, occasionally in conjunction with a bicuspid or absent pulmonary valve. Partial or complete atrioventricular canal defects form a spectrum of abnormally formed leaflets. Subaortic stenosis is recognizable by hypoplasia or hyperkinesis of the aortic conus. Extracardiac anomalies abound and include anomalous pulmonary venous connection, bilateral superior vena cava, patent ductus arteriosus, coarctation and interruption of the aortic arch, and the heterotaxy syndrome.

The angiographic evaluation of double-outlet right ventricle necessitates biplane right and left ventriculograms. Simultaneous opacification of both great arteries after a ventriculogram is a typical feature of this malformation, but one artery may fill before the other when premature

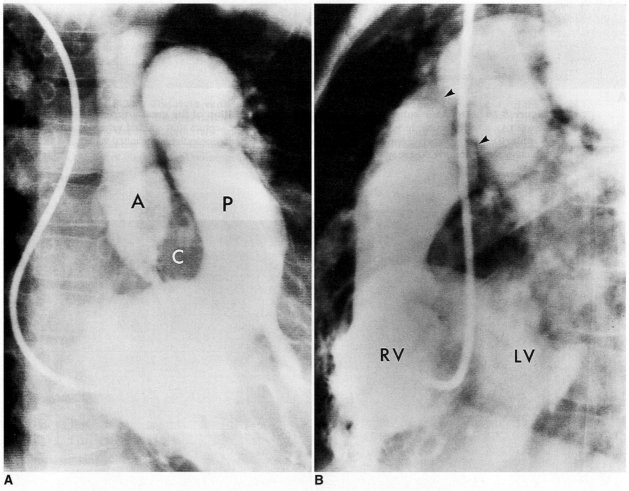

A   **B**

Figure 8-28   Angiographic features of double-outlet right ventricle. A, In the frontal projection, the aorta originates adjacent to the ventricular septal defect. Severe subaortic stenosis narrows the outflow tract to a few millimeters. The crista supraventricularis (C) is common to both the subaortic and subpulmonary conus. **B,** In the lateral view, the left ventricle (LV) is opacified through a large ventricular septal defect. The aorta is not visualized, as it lies beside and is obscured by the large pulmonary artery. A loose pulmonary band (arrowheads) is present. A, aorta; P, pulmonary artery; RV, right ventricle.

ventricular contractions occur or when there is subpulmonary or subaortic stenosis.

If double-outlet right ventricle is suspected, angiography in the posteroanterior and lateral views identifies the position of the aorta and pulmonary artery. The angled oblique views, particularly the left ventriculogram, show the abnormalities in the atrioventricular valves and the location and size of the ventricular septal defect. The plane of the ventricular septum is in the normal left anterior oblique projection in those hearts in situs solitus and D-loop ventricles. If there are inverted ventricles, the typical ventricular septum is sagittal and therefore aligned on the posteroanterior view.

There are many angiographic features characteristic of double-outlet right ventricle in situs solitus (Fig. 8-28). In the frontal view, the heavily trabeculated right ventricle partially overlies the posterior left ventricle. Both semilunar valves have the same height and are separated from the rest of the heart by a bilateral conus. The central lucency between the aortic and pulmonary outflow tracts is the crista supraventricularis. On the lateral view, there is discontinuity between the atrioventricular valves and the semilunar valves. Behind the great arteries and the mitral valve there is a notch that represents the ventriculo-infundibular recess. The conus under both great arteries generally overlaps completely so that, unless one artery fills before the other, the relation of the conus to the ventricle may be difficult to recognize. In the uncommon Taussig–Bing type of double-outlet right ventricle (Fig. 8-29), the pulmonary artery is adjacent to the ventricular septal defect.

Pulmonary stenosis (Fig. 8-30), both the subvalvular and valvular varieties, exists in about half of patients with double-outlet right ventricle. Conversely, subaortic stenosis occurs in about 20% of patients with this defect. Since the semilunar valves tend to lie on a transaxial plane, nonangled films in the frontal plane project the annulus of both the aortic and pulmonary valves in tangent. An injection in the outflow tract or directly beneath the crista supraventricularis may aid in making these outflow obstructions visible. (Table 8-4 illustrates the differential diagnosis of double-outlet right ventricle.)

Double-outlet Left Ventricle

Double-outlet left ventricle is a rare type of partial transposition. In its complete form, both the aorta and pulmonary artery connect above the left ventricle. This malformation has one great artery and half of the other great artery arising above the left ventricle. Since this classification involves only the ventriculoarterial relations, it is not surprising that double-outlet left ventricle comprises a heterogeneous group of malformations that are associated with multiple anomalies and malpositions of the atrioventricular segments. Anomalies associated with double-outlet left ventricle are:

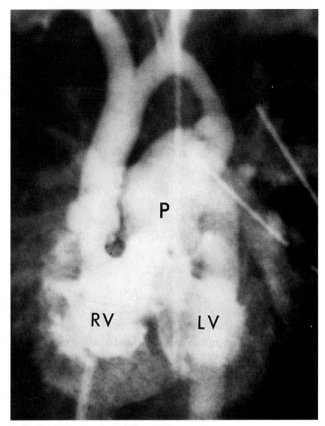

Figure 8-29   Taussig–Bing malformation. In this double-outlet right ventricle (RV), a small bilateral conus is present with moderate subaortic stenosis. The pulmonary artery (P) originates above the ventricular septal defect. An aortic coarctation is associated with mild hypoplasia of the arch. The large ventricular septal defect is the only outlet of the left ventricle (LV).

- stenosis or atresia of any of the four cardiac valves
- preductal coarctation
- patent ductus arteriosus
- Ebstein's anomaly
- situs inversus.

Most hearts with this malformation have a bilaterally absent conus, although there may be a subpulmonary or subaortic conus.

Table 8-4	Differential Diagnosis of Double-outlet Right Ventricle	
Findings in Double-outlet Right Ventricle	**Alternative Findings**	**Alternative Diagnosis**
Bilateral conus	Pulmonary mitral continuity	Transposition of great arteries
	Aortic–mitral continuity	Tetralogy of Fallot

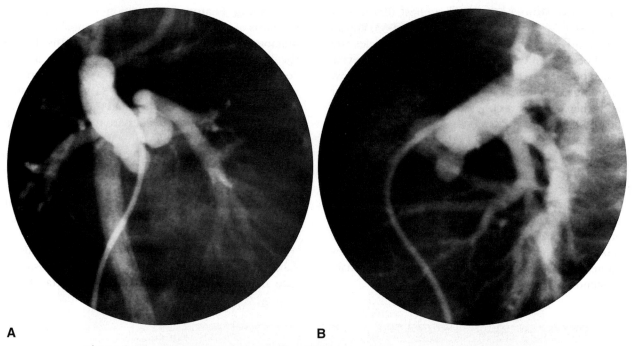

A   **B**

Figure 8-35   Truncus arteriosus. A, The right anterior oblique truncal arteriogram shows the right aortic arch with mirror-image branching. **B,** The lateral view shows a tricuspid truncal valve without regurgitation. The pulmonary arteries originate posteriorly from the truncus.

types A1 and A2 may be difficult to distinguish when the main pulmonary artery is short. Steep cranially angled views may be helpful. Selective angiography of each pulmonary artery may visualize their origins by backward reflux. Angiography in type A3 shows only one pulmonary artery arising from the truncus; the other lung is supplied by collaterals from the descending aorta. If the left pulmonary artery is not visible following ventricular or truncal injections, you should perform aortography with the catheter at the aortic isthmus to search for the left pulmonary artery. You may recognize type A4 truncus on a ventriculogram as a small ascending aorta that comes from the right anterolateral aspect of the pulmonary artery. It may be difficult to identify whether the catheter has passed around the aortic arch or through a patent ductus arteriosus.

Magnetic resonance imaging can provide a valuable adjunct to angiography and echocardiography by non-invasively locating the mediastinal pulmonary arteries (Fig. 8-36). Spin-echo images are obtained in the coronal and axial planes for the origins of the pulmonary arteries. Small arteries near the lung border are better identified with flow sequences such as cine gradient-recalled techniques or phase reconstruction.

Hemitruncus Arteriosus

In hemitruncus one of the pulmonary arteries originates from the aorta and the other from the right ventricle.

There are separate aortic and pulmonary valves which distinguish hemitruncus from truncus type A3. The lung connected to the aorta is subject to the systemic pressure and has aneurysmal hilar branches and serpentine peripheral vessels. The lung supplied by the right ventricle has normal vasculature. The aortic arch tends to be large and may displace the trachea away from the side of the arch. It is right-sided in 20–30% of cases. When the thymus does not obscure the mediastinum, the right boundary is the edge of the large ascending aorta.

Large patent ductus arteriosus, tetralogy of Fallot with pulmonary atresia, and aortopulmonary septation are the other major cardiac anomalies to be differentiated from truncus arteriosus. If two semilunar valves are identified, the diagnosis is not truncus. To make this distinction it may take injections in both right and left ventricles, particularly since a ventricular septal defect is also present in all these malformations. A blind infundibular chamber in the right ventricle is typical of tetralogy of Fallot with pulmonary atresia. During right ventriculography in the lateral projection, this chamber is seen as an outpouching anterior to the aorta; this chamber is not present in truncus arteriosus.

Aortopulmonary Septation

Separate aortic and pulmonary valves and a defect between the ascending aorta and the main or right pulmonary artery are characteristic of aortopulmonary

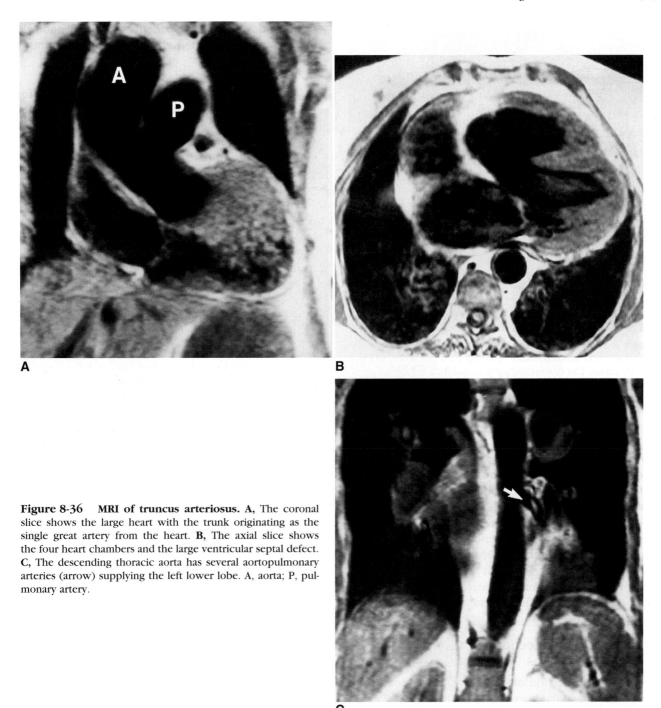

Figure 8-36   MRI of truncus arteriosus. A, The coronal slice shows the large heart with the trunk originating as the single great artery from the heart. **B,** The axial slice shows the four heart chambers and the large ventricular septal defect. **C,** The descending thoracic aorta has several aortopulmonary arteries (arrow) supplying the left lower lobe. A, aorta; P, pulmonary artery.

septation (Fig. 8-37). This rare malformation is also called aortopulmonary septal defect and aortic pulmonary window. The defect is usually in the left lateral wall of the ascending aorta and connects with the right lateral wall of the pulmonary trunk. The defect can extend from the annulus of the two semilunar valves to involve the ascending aorta to varying degrees. About half have aortic arch interruption or a preductile coarctation.

Anatomically Corrected Malposition of the Great Arteries
In this malformation, the left ventricle ejects into the aorta and the right ventricle into the pulmonary artery.

and systemic circulation, and the degree of pulmonary vascular obstruction. Most of these patients have either an atrial septal defect or patent foramen ovale, which serves as the conduit to the systemic circulation. The blood flow is bidirectional at the right atrium, passing either into the left atrium or into the right ventricle and pulmonary artery. Increased pulmonary blood flow occurs in the supracardiac and cardiac level anomalies. Decreased pulmonary blood flow can, of course, occur from an Eisenmenger reaction with an increase in the precapillary vascular resistance. In the infracardiac type, the pulmonary venous return is obstructed mainly by the portal circulation. The physiologic consequences are signs of pulmonary venous hypertension and pulmonary edema.

Chest Film Findings. The findings on the chest film depend on the same variables that control the blood flow to the heart and lungs. When there is no pulmonary venous obstruction, typically in the supracardiac and intracardiac types, the chest film generally demonstrates cardiomegaly and large pulmonary vessels. The right atrial and ventricular contours appear prominent, and there is no evidence of left atrial enlargement, even on the barium esophagogram. The right superior vena cava is dilated when it is part of the circuit that receives

pulmonary venous drainage. The only sign pathognomonic of the supracardiac variety that is seen on the chest film is the 'snowman' configuration (Fig. 8-39). The anomalous left vertical vein forms the convex left superior mediastinal border as it joins the dilated left innominate vein. The enlarged right superior vena cava protrudes into the right lung, completing the head of the snowman.

In those cases that are obstructive, the chest film is quite different (Fig. 8-40). Generally, the heart is of normal size without prominence of any chamber. The striking abnormality occurs in the lungs, which show evidence of pulmonary edema. An interstitial pattern is invariably present in the infracardiac type. Interstitial and alveolar pulmonary edema and, occasionally, Kerley B lines are frequently mistaken for noncardiac causes of pulmonary consolidation, such as neonatal pneumonia, aspiration, respiratory distress syndrome, and transient tachypnea of the newborn.

The angiographic technique for identifying the course and location of the anomalous veins begins with pulmonary arteriography. In the supracardiac variety with the anomalous left vertical vein, the vein itself may be injected directly. In the newborn, this structure may be fragile so that indirect opacification from a more

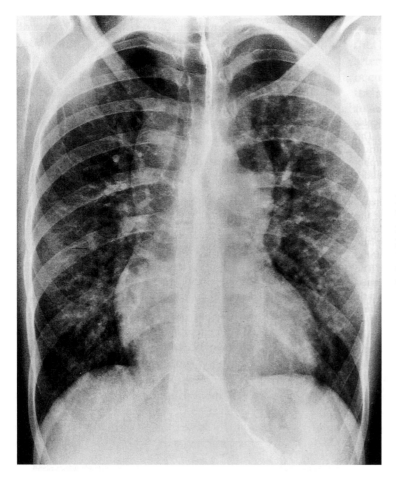

Figure 8-39   Chest film in supracardiac type of total anomalous pulmonary venous connection. The pulmonary vessels are large, consistent with increased pulmonary blood flow. The abnormal mediastinum (the 'snowman') is caused by the dilated right superior vena cava on the right side and by the anomalous vertical vein draining both lungs on the left side.

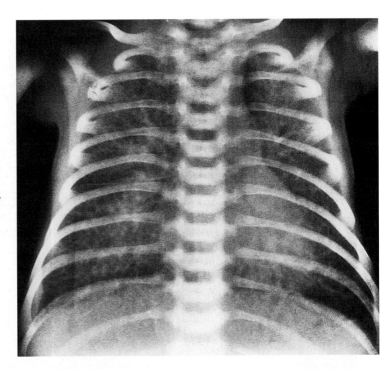

Figure 8-40   Chest film in total anomalous pulmonary venous connection to the portal vein. The small heart size reflects the diminished inflow to the left side of the heart through an atrial septal defect. Pulmonary edema and a small heart are sentinel features of the infracardiac type of total anomalous pulmonary venous connection.

peripheral site is desirable. A main pulmonary artery angiogram in the posteroanterior projection demonstrates the pulmonary veins on the levophase (Fig. 8-41). In the lateral view, the confluence of veins appears behind the usual position of the left atrium before it ascends into the anomalous vertical vein to join the left innominate vein. If other cardiac defects are discovered, additional injections will clarify their morphology.

In the intracardiac type, the location of the anomalous connection may be difficult to identify because of overlapping cardiac chambers. Pulmonary angiography with late filming for the levophase structures shows opacification of the coronary sinus or right atrium before the left atrium (Fig. 8-42).

The infracardiac variety is distinctive and has considerably reduced blood flow (Fig. 8-43). For this reason,

Figure 8-41   Total anomalous venous connection to vertical vein. Levophase of pulmonary angiogram in the anteroposterior projection shows all pulmonary veins connecting behind the left atrium to form an anomalous vertical vein. This structure forms the left mediastinal border and joins the left innominate vein. The right superior vena cava is dilated and occupies the right side of the mediastinum.

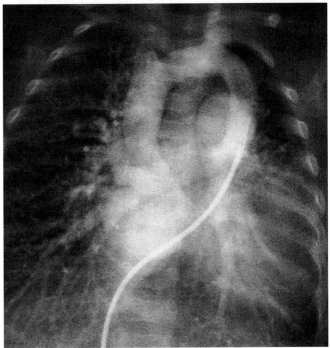

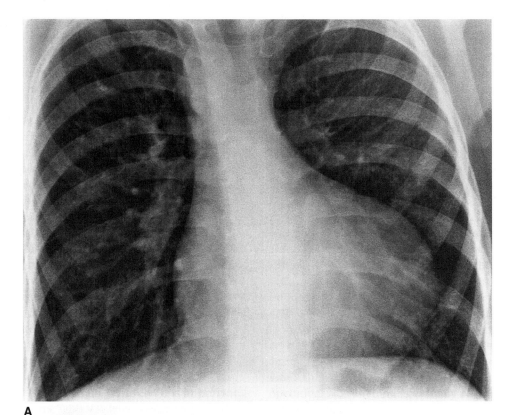

A

B

Figure 8-76 Tetralogy of Fallot in the adult. A, The heart is mildly enlarged with an uplifted apex. The main pulmonary artery segment is straight and the hilar arteries are slightly small. The aortic arch is right-sided. **B,** Moderate pulmonary stenosis, moderate pulmonary hypertension, and a bidirectional ventricular shunt are atypical features of tetralogy in this cyanotic 67-year-old man. Note the differential size of the peripheral right and left pulmonary arteries. Large internal mammary artery collaterals (arrow) connect to the hila.

the diaphragm, and hyperaerated lungs may interpose between the heart and diaphragm.

You can usually ascertain the side of the aortic arch on the frontal chest film when you cannot see the tracheal air column. In neonates, the trachea buckles away from the side of the arch on expiration. In children and adults, the side of the arch is determined in the usual fashion by the asymmetry of tissue at the level of the aortic arch. When a right aortic arch is suspected, cross-sectional imaging can be helpful. An isolated right aortic arch with a normal heart has a retroesophageal left subclavian artery; the esophagus is deviated anteriorly by the anomalous left subclavian artery. In over 96% of instances of right aortic arch associated with tetralogy of Fallot, there is no retroesophageal anomalous artery. The branching pattern of the aortic arch is then a mirror image of the normal left aortic arch; that is, the order of vessels is the left innominate artery, the right carotid artery, and the right subclavian artery.

Angiographic Examination

The ventricular septal defect is best seen on the left anterior oblique projection with cranial angulation (long-axis

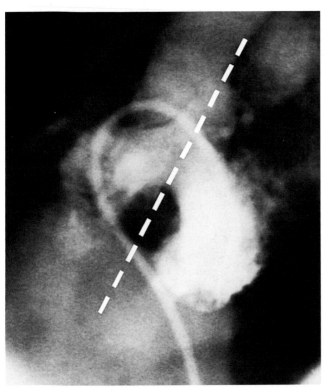

Figure 8-77 Overriding aorta in tetralogy of Fallot. A left ventriculogram in the cranial left anterior oblique projection was performed with the catheter going through a patent foramen ovale. A line drawn through the interventricular septum locates most of the aortic valve over the right ventricle. In the normal heart, there is less than 25% aortic overriding.

oblique view) so as not to foreshorten the ventricular septum. With either a right or left ventricular injection, the ventricular septal defect can be seen extending from the aortic valve inferiorly to the muscular ventricular septum (Fig. 8-77). The malalignment of the infundibular septum with the aorta and pulmonary trunk projects the parietal band anteriorly and differentiates this type of ventricular septal defect from a membranous septal defect. In the left anterior oblique projection, the aortic valve straddles or overrides the ventricular septum to quite a variable degree. Follow the plane of the interventricular septum as it intersects the aortic valve to measure the amount of overriding. The following associated defects that are important to evaluate are best visualized in the cranial left anterior oblique view:

- position and size of ventricular septal defects
- morphology of infundibular and valvular pulmonary stenosis
- hypoplasia or atresia of the pulmonary arteries
- confluence of the pulmonary arteries across the midline
- aortic mitral separation to distinguish from double-outlet right ventricle
- aberrant left coronary artery from the right coronary artery
- right- or left-sided aortic arch
- atrioventricular canal defect.

Visualization of the bifurcation of the main pulmonary artery is best accomplished by right ventriculography with 40° of cranial angulation in the posteroanterior projection or in the hepatoclavicular view (40° cranial and 40° left anterior). These views place the pulmonary valve, main pulmonary artery, and both central branches in the same plane, perpendicular to the x-ray beam (Fig. 8-78). When pulmonary atresia is present, selective catheterization of the bronchial and intercostal arteries that supply the lungs may show the location of all the pulmonary blood supply. The right and left pulmonary arteries may not connect across the mediastinum. In the older child and adult, MRI is an excellent modality to search for small mediastinal arteries. Although spin-echo images are usually diagnostic, the imaging of small pulmonary arteries and aortopulmonary collaterals may require flow-sensitive techniques.

Approximately 5% of patients with tetralogy of Fallot have surgically important coronary anomalies. The most common major anomaly is the origin of the left anterior descending artery from the right coronary artery. In this anomaly, the aberrant artery courses over the usual site of infundibulotomy. The surgeon attempts to avoid transecting the anterior descending artery in this location because a major left ventricular infarction would usually result. In infants, the coronary arteries are visualized by aortography, by passing the transvenous catheter into the aortic root from the right ventricle and ventricular

Didier D, Ratib O, Beghetti M, *et al.* Morphologic and functional evaluation of congenital heart disease by magnetic resonance imaging. *J Magn Reson Imaging* 1999;10:639.

Dinsmore RE, Wismer GL, Guyer D, *et al.* Magnetic resonance imaging of the interatrial septum and atrial septal defects. *AJR* 1985;145:697.

Dotter CT, Steinberg I. Angiocardiography in congenital heart disease. *Am J Med* 1952;12:219.

Elliott LP. *Cardiac imaging in infants, children, and adults.* Philadelphia: JB Lippincott, 1991.

Emmanouilides GC, Riemenschneider TA, Allen HD, *et al. Moss and Adams heart disease in infants, children, and adolescents including the fetus and young adults,* 6th ed. Baltimore, MD: Williams & Wilkins, 2000.

Farre JR. *Pathological researches. Essay I. On malformations of the heart.* London: Longman, Hurst, Rees, Orme & Brown, 1814:28.

Figley MM. Accessory roentgen signs of coarctation of the aorta. *Radiology* 1954;62:671.

Freedom RM, Benson LN, Smallhorn JF. *Neonatal heart disease.* London: Springer-Verlag, 1992.

Freedom RM, Culham JAG, Moes CAF. *Angiocardiography of congenital heart disease.* New York: Macmillan, 1997.

Fulcher AS, Turner MA. Abdominal manifestations of situs anomalies in adults. *RadioGraphics* 2002;22:1439.

Gross GW, Steiner RM. Radiographic manifestations of congenital heart disease in the adult patient. *Radiol Clin North Am* 1991;29:103.

Higgins CB, Silverman NH, Kersting-Sommerhoff BA, *et al. Congenital heart disease. Echocardiography and magnetic resonance imaging.* New York: Raven Press, 1990.

Hoffman JIE, Kaplan S. Incidence of congenital heart disease. *J Am Coll Radiol* 2002;39:12.

Ivemark BI. Implications of agenesis of the spleen on the pathogenesis of contruncus anomalies in childhood: an analysis of the heart; malformations in the splenic agenesis syndrome, with fourteen new cases. *Acta Paediatr Scand Suppl* 1966;104:1.

Jaffe RB. Complete interruption of the aortic arch: 1. Characteristic of radiographic findings in 21 patients. *Circulation* 1975;52:714.

Jaffe RB. Complete interruption of the aortic arch: 2. Characteristic angiographic features with emphasis on collateral circulation to the descending aorta. *Circulation* 1976;53:161.

Jaffe RB, Scherer JL. Supracristal ventricular septal defects: spectrum of associated lesions and complications. *AJR* 1977; 128:629.

Kersting-Sommerhoff BA, Seelos KC, Hardy C, *et al.* Evaluation of surgical procedures for cyanotic congenital heart disease by using MR imaging. *AJR,* 1990;155:259.

Kiely B, Filler J, Stone S, *et al.* Syndrome of anomalous venous drainage of the right lung to the inferior vena cava. A review of 67 reported cases and three new cases in children. *Am J Cardiol* 1967;20:102.

Landing BH, Lawrence TK, Payne VC Jr, *et al.* Bronchial anatomy in syndromes with abnormal visceral situs, abnormal spleen and congenital heart disease. *Am J Cardiol* 1971; 28:456.

Lavin N, Mehta S, Liberson M, *et al.* Pseudocoarctation of the aorta: an unusual variant with coarctation. *Am J Cardiol* 1969;24:584.

Liberthson RR, Pennington DG, Jacobs M, *et al.* Coarctation of the aorta: review of 234 patients and clarification of management problems. *Am J Cardiol* 1979;43:835.

McCartney JF, Shinebourne EA, Anderson RH. Connexions, relations, discordance, and distortions. *Br Heart J* 1976; 38:323.

Midiri M, Finazzo M, Di Francesco M, *et al.* Congenitally corrected transposition of great vessels: MRI and echocardiographic appearance. *Eur J Radiol* 1995;5:672.

Neye-Bock S, Fellows KE. Aortic arch interruption in infancy: radio- and angiographic features. *AJR* 1980;135:1005.

Partridge JB, Scott O, Deverall PB, *et al.* Visualization and measurement of the main bronchi by tomography as an objective indicator of thoracic situs in congenital heart disease. *Circulation* 1975;51:188.

Patterson W, Baxley WA, Karp RB, *et al.* Tricuspid atresia in adults. *Am J Cardiol* 1982;49:141.

Perloff JK, Child JS. Congenital heart disease in adults. Philadelphia, PA: WB Saunders, 1998.

Piccoli GP, Gerlis LM, Wilkinson JL, *et al.* Morphology and classification of atrioventricular defects. *Br Heart J* 1979; 42:621.

Randall PA, Moller JH, Amplatz K. The spleen and congenital heart disease. *AJR* 1973;119:551.

Rao PS. A unified classification for tricuspid atresia. *Am Heart J* 1980;99:799.

Rao PS. Dextrocardia: systematic approach to differential diagnosis. *Am Heart J* 1981;102:389.

Rose V, Izukawa T, Moes CAF. Syndromes of asplenia and polysplenia. A review of cardiac and non-cardiac malformations in 60 cases with special reference to diagnosis and prognosis. *Br Heart J* 1975;37:840.

Rothko K, Moore GW, Hutchins GM. Truncus arteriosus malformation: a spectrum including fourth and sixth aortic arch interruptions. *Am Heart J* 1980;99:17.

Shinebourne EA, Macartney FJ, Anderson RH. Sequential chamber localization – logical approach to diagnosis in congenital heart disease. *Br Heart J* 1976;38:327.

Shinebourne EA, Lau KC, Calcaterra G, *et al.* Univentricular heart or right ventricular type: clinical, angiographic and electrocardiographic features. *Am J Cardiol* 1980;46:439.

Sloan RD, Cooley RN. Coarctation of the aorta. The roentgenologic aspects of one hundred and twenty-five surgically confirmed cases. *Radiology* 1953;61:701.

Smyth PT, Edwards JE. Pseudocoarctation, kinking or buckling of the aorta. *Circulation* 1972;46:1027.

Soto B, Bargeron LM Jr, Paacifico AD, *et al.* Angiography of atrioventricular canal defects. *Am J Cardiol* 1981;48:492.

Soto B, Becker AE, Moulaert AJ, *et al.* Classification of ventricular septal defects. *Br Heart J* 1980;43:332.

Soto B, Bertranou EG, Bream PR, *et al.* Angiographic study of univentricular heart of right ventricular type. *Circulation* 1979; 60:1325.

Soto B, Pacifico AS, Souza AD, *et al.* Identification of thoracic isomerism from the plain chest radiograph. *AJR* 1978; 131:995.

Soto B, Pacifico AD. Angiocardiography in congenital heart malformations. Mount Kisco, NY: Futura, 1990.

Stanger P, Rudolph AM, Edwards JE. Cardiac malpositions. An overview based on study of sixty-five necropsy specimens. *Circulation* 1977;56:159.

Swischuk LE. Differential diagnosis in pediatric radiology. Baltimore, MD: Williams & Wilkins, 1994.

Taussig HB. Tetralogy of Fallot: early history and late results. *AJR* 1979;133:423.

Tonkin ID. Pediatric cardiovascular imaging. Philadelphia, PA: WB Saunders, 1992.

Van Mierop LHS, Eisen S, Schiebler GL. The radiographic appearance of the tracheobronchial tree as an indicator of visceral situs. *Am J Cardiol* 1970;25:432.

Van Praagh R. Terminology of congenital heart disease. Glossary and commentary (editorial). *Circulation* 1977;56:139.

Van Praagh R. What is the Taussig–Bing malformation? (editorial). *Circulation* 1968;38:445.

Van Praagh R, Van Praagh S. Isolated ventricular inversion. A consideration of the morphogenesis, definition and diagnosis of nontransposed and transposed great arteries. *Am J Cardiol* 1966;17:395.

Van Praagh R, Van Praagh S, Vlad P, *et al.* Anatomic types of congenital dextrocardia. Diagnostic and embryologic implications. *Am J Cardiol* 1964;13:510.

Van Praagh R, Van Praagh S, Nebesar RA, *et al.* Tetralogy of Fallot: underdevelopment of the pulmonary infundibulum and its sequelae. *Am J Cardiol* 1970;26:25.

Van Praagh R, Durnin RE, Jockin H, *et al.* Anatomically corrected malposition of the great arteries (S,D,L). *Circulation* 1975;51:20.

Van Praagh R, Papagiannis J, Grunefleder J, *et al.* Pathologic anatomy of corrected transposition of the great arteries: medical and surgical implications. *Am Heart J* 1998;135:772.

Van Praagh R, Van Praagh S, Vlad P, *et al.* Diagnosis of the anatomic types of single or common ventricle. *Am J Cardiol* 15:345, 1965.

Wilkinson JL, Acerete F. Terminological pitfalls in congenital heart disease. Reappraisal of some confusing terms, with an account of a simplified system of basic nomenclature. *Br Heart J* 1973;35:1166.

Wimpftheimer O, Bac LM. MR imaging of adult patients with congenital heart disease. *Radiol Clin North Am* 1999;37:421.

Winer-Muram HT, Tonkin ILD. The spectrum of heterotaxic syndromes. *Radiol Clin North Am* 1989;27:1147.

Woodring JH, Howard TA, Kanga JF. Congenital pulmonary venolobar syndrome. *Radiographics* 1994;14:349.

Marfan syndrome. Cardiomegaly is usually nonspecific and may reflect only the pectus excavatum, but aortic regurgitation from annuloaortic ectasia and mitral regurgitation from prolapsing mitral leaflets are common conditions that pathologically enlarge the heart. On the lateral film, a pectus excavatum is frequently identified as well as a narrow thoracic diameter.

Marfan patients without symptoms are easily observed with serial MRI every 6–12 months. Surgical referral is usually undertaken if a previously stable aortic aneurysm begins to enlarge or if the aortic arch and descending aorta exceed a diameter of 5 cm. MRI allows detection of the onset of annuloaortic ectasia (Figure 9-19) with dilatation of the aortic root and ascending aorta, as well as visualization of a dissection. Aortic regurgitation can be observed and quantified with velocity-encoded pulse sequences. Observations on the aortic root and quantification of aortic regurgitation can also be made by echocardiography.

Aortography is usually reserved for urgent clinical situations where noninvasive imaging was inconclusive. Some surgeons request coronary angiography to evaluate whether a dissection extends near or into the coronary arteries. Occasionally, aortography can identify an entry site of a dissection that is not apparent on other methods (Figure 9-20).

Sinus of Valsalva Aneurysms

Etiology

Dilatation of one or all of the sinuses of Valsalva may be associated with abnormalities in the aortic valve or the aorta. These aneurysms may be classified radiologically as discrete (localized to the sinuses) or annuloaortic (involving both the aortic root and the ascending aorta). The classic type is annuloaortic ectasia with a pear-shaped configuration of the aortic root and equal dilatation of all sinuses.

An outline of sinus of Valsalva aneurysms is presented in Box 9-4. Discrete aneurysms that involve a single sinus are usually congenital (Figure 9-21), although rarely dilatation of two or all three sinuses may also be congenital. These are generally less than 4 cm in diameter and involve mainly the right sinus. The tissue in the aortic annulus adjacent to the leaflet histologically has sparse fibroelastic elements and grossly may have fenestrations through the cusp. A sinus of Valsalva aneurysm can develop as a consequence of a ventricular septal defect. One of the ways a ventricular septal defect can close spontaneously is to form fibrous tissue around its edges. As the membranous ventricular septal defect becomes smaller, the adjacent leaflet of the aortic valve is pulled inferiorly into the defect. The clinical consequence of the developing leaflet prolapse is that the left-to-right shunt

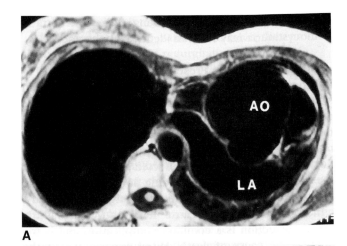

A

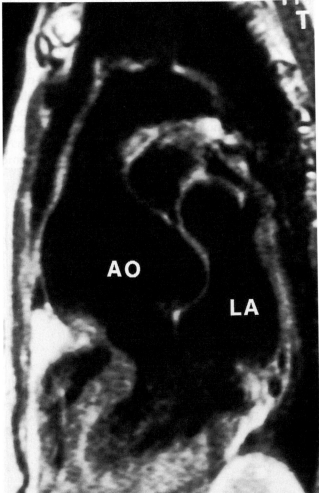

B

Figure 9-19   MR image in annuloaortic ectasia. A, The thorax has a narrow anteroposterior diameter with a mild pectus excavatum. The aortic root (AO) is huge and occupies a major portion of the left hemithorax in front of the left atrium (LA). **B,** A sagittal plane shows the loss of the sinotubular ridge as the aneurysm extends from the sinuses of Valsalva to half of the ascending aorta. The left atrium is quite dilated.

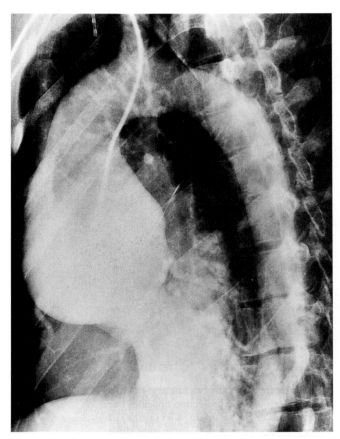

Figure 9-20   Annuloaortic ectasia. The aneurysm involves both the sinuses of Valsalva and the proximal half of the ascending aorta. The dilatation of the annulus has secondarily caused aortic regurgitation. The left ventricle is enlarged and is densely opacified, indicating a severe degree of insufficiency.

Box 9-4   Sinus of Valsalva Aneurysms

Congenital: Single cusp involved with normal aorta
   Localized deficiency of the tissue in the aortic annulus
   Retraction of a cusp into a closing ventricular septal defect
Inherited: All cusps involved with annuloaortic ectasia
   Marfan syndrome
   Ehlers: Danlos syndrome
Acquired: Saccular false aneurysms
   Aortic root abscess with endocarditis
   Luetic aortitis
   Aortic dissection

---

through the ventricular septal defect is transformed to that of aortic regurgitation.

Acquired discrete aneurysms usually involve all three sinuses if they are a consequence of a generalized inflammatory process, for example, syphilis or an immune complex aortitis. Aortic root abscesses are actually false aneurysms since they erode through the aorta into cardiac or mediastinal tissue.

Since the sinuses of Valsalva lie completely within the cardiac silhouette (Figure 9-22), the discrete type of aneurysm is not visible on the plain chest film. If the ascending aorta is also dilated, the right side of the mediastinum will have the characteristic convexity of the aorta as it extends into the adjacent lung.

Calcification

Calcification of the sinuses of Valsalva above the aortic leaflets is rare. If there is also extensive aortic calcification, this indicates syphilitic aortitis. Mild calcification of the nondilated sinuses and flecks in the ascending aorta suggest the presence of type II hyperlipoproteinemia. Rarely, congenital or nonsyphilitic aneurysms in the aortic root may calcify.

Complications

Aortic regurgitation is the main complication of progressive dilatation of the aortic annulus and the resultant lack of coaptation of the leaflets. Any type of sinus of Valsalva aneurysm can rupture into an adjacent structure. The onset is abrupt with severe aortic regurgitation or a torrential left-to-right shunt. Most sinus aneurysms rupture into the right sinus; they perforate anteriorly into the right ventricular outflow tract, dissect into the ventricular septum, or perforate posteriorly in the right atrium. Aneurysms of the noncoronary sinus rupture into the right atrium. Rupture of the left sinus into the left atrial appendage is extremely rare. When an aneurysm ruptures, aortography shows contrast medium entering the cardiac chamber and opacifying downstream structures on subsequent films (Figure 9-23). Both a left ventriculogram and an aortogram may be necessary to distinguish a ventricular septal defect with aortic regurgitation from a ruptured sinus of Valsalva aneurysm. The contrast in the right ventricle from an aortogram could have passed into the left ventricle from aortic regurgitation and then across a ventricular septal defect, or it could have flowed directly from the aorta through the rupture into the right ventricle.

Since an aneurysm of the right sinus of Valsalva can compress and distort adjacent structures, significant hemodynamic complications can occur as the aneurysm dilates. Right coronary artery compression, superior vena cava obstruction, right ventricular outflow obstruction, and endocarditis can produce dramatic clinical events.

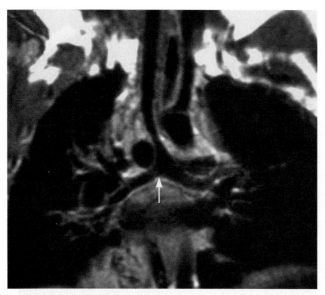

Figure 9-64   Pulmonary sling. Coronal MRI demonstrating stretching of the right main stem bronchus (arrow) by the left pulmonary artery. (Courtesy of Laureen Sena, M.D.)

artery from the aorta occurs in tetralogy of Fallot with right aortic arch.

Coarctation of the Aorta

In 1791 Paris delivered a paper on the pathology of coarctation. Although the clinical and pathologic signs of collateral flow in coarctation were known in the 19th century, the radiologic recognition of rib notching and the abnormal mediastinal silhouette were not firmly established until nearly 30 years after the first chest films were taken. In 1928, Abbott described the rib notching from enlarged intercostal vessels and the size discrepancy between the aortic arch and the descending aorta at the level of the left subclavian artery. Some of the first angiographic examinations were performed for coarctation in 1941.

Imaging Diagnosis

In current medical practice, the diagnosis of coarctation that is suggested on physical examination is confirmed by imaging. The chest film in the adult frequently shows the notched aortic isthmus, but this sign is usually not seen in the infant. In infants, the evaluation of coarctation is typically made by echocardiography. In children and adults, MRI and occasionally angiography provide additional important information and may modify the medical and surgical management. These additional observations include associated aortic arch anomalies, aberrant subclavian vessels, atypical or long-segment aortic stenoses, and patent ductus arteriosus. At times, abundant collaterals that are evident on angiography

were undetected by the physical examination or the chest film. When minimal collaterals are present, the surgical approach may change from a primary repair to a bypass graft around the coarctation in order to protect the blood supply to the spinal canal.

Classification

There are numerous classifications of coarctation based on the age of the patient, the position of a patent ductus arteriosus in relation to the coarctation, and the length of the coarctation. Most of these schemata, including the classification into infantile or adult types, have limited usefulness in patient management because there is great variability within the categories, and the adult type of coarctation is frequently present in infants. Preductal and postductal coarctation are meaningful if the ductus is patent. Box 9-8 is a useful list of imaging observations that includes ductal patency, extent of collaterals, aortic arch anomalies, and coarctation in unusual locations.

Characteristics

The typical coarctation occurs in the aortic isthmus. This segment of the aorta between the origin of the left subclavian artery and the ductus is normally slightly small in the fetus and newborn. The fetal configuration of the isthmus produces a diameter that is roughly three-quarters of the diameter of the descending thoracic aorta. Three months after birth, the fetal configuration of the isthmus is gone and the aortic arch has the same diameter throughout. The coarctation consists of an obstructing membrane on the greater curvature of the aorta opposite the ductus or ligamentum arteriosum. Typically, the lesser curvature of the aorta, which includes the site of the ductus, is retracted medially toward the left pulmonary artery. Beyond the obstruction there is usually a short segment that is dilated and may rarely be aneurysmal. The aorta proximal to the coarctation may be enlarged, either congenitally or from hypertension. The dilatation may include the innominate, carotid, and subclavian vessels. More than half have tubular hypoplasia of the transverse portion of the aortic arch, beginning after the innominate artery and ending at the coarctation. In this configuration, the innominate, carotid, and subclavian arteries are dilated and may be as large as the transverse aortic arch.

The position of a patent ductus arteriosus with respect to the coarctation affects both the clinical presentation and the imaging interpretation. A ductus arteriosus may originate proximal, distal, or adjacent to a coarctation. If the coarctation is distal to the ductus arteriosus, blood flow is initially from the aorta to the pulmonary arteries in a left-to-right direction. If later the pulmonary vascular resistance increases because of an Eisenmenger reaction, the shunt may become bidirectional or reversed. If the coarctation is proximal to the ductus arteriosus, flow

Box 9-8 Imaging Evaluation of Coarctation of the Aorta

PATENCY OF THE DUCTUS ARTERIOSUS

Closed

Patent
- Flow from aorta to pulmonary artery (typically postductal coarctation)
- Flow from pulmonary artery to aorta (preductal coarctation or pulmonary hypertension

COLLATERAL PATHWAYS

Scarce (typical of patients under 2 years of age)

Abundant
- Bridging the coarctated segment
- Internal mammary to intercostal to distal aorta
- Circumscapular pathyways to distal aorta

OTHER ARCH ANOMALIES AND STENOSES

Arch interruption

Double aortic arch with stenosis in either or both arches

Coarctation proximal to left subclavian artery

Takayasu's aortitis, rubella, Williams syndrome, neurofibromatosis, mucopolysaccharidosis, and other causes of stenoses not in the aortic isthmus

SUBCLAVIAN ARTERY ANOMALIES

Atresia or stenosis of the left subclavian artery

Aberrant retroesophageal right subclavian artery
- Proximal to the coarctation
- Distal to the coarcation

Origin of both subclavian arteries distal to the coarctation

ASSOCIATED LESIONS

Cardiac, such as ventricular septal defect or bicuspid aortic valve

Aneurysms
- In aorta adjacent to coarctation
- In the ductus
- In the intercostal arteries
- In the circle of Willis

Stenosis or the anomalous origin of a subclavian artery distal to the coarctation results in an inequality in pulses and blood pressures in the two arms. A rare condition that produces equal blood pressures in both arms is the anomalous origin of both subclavian arteries below the coarctation. Coarctation at multiple sites or in the distal thoracic and abdominal aorta probably represents an embryologically different malformation such as neurofibromatosis, or an acquired disease such as Takayasu's aortoarteritis. Mucopolysaccharidosis (Hurler and Scheie syndromes) may have long tubular segmental stenoses in the aorta resembling those seen in Takayasu's disease.

Congenital bicuspid aortic valve is frequently associated with coarctation. Between a quarter and half of the patients with aortic coarctation also have a bicuspid aortic valve. Anomalies associated with aortic coarctation are listed in Box 9-9.

Fatal complications of aortic coarctation include bacterial aortitis at the site of the coarctation, aortic dissection, aneurysm of the ductus with rupture, and distal thromboembolism. Fatal left ventricular failure may occur from hypertensive heart disease or from stenosis and regurgitation of a bicuspid aortic valve. Since the carotid arteries are hypertensive, aneurysms in the circle of Willis may develop and rupture.

Chest Film Abnormalities

Plain film findings have their angiographic counterpart and are particularly useful in searching for the extent of collateral supply. The thoracic aorta shows an abnormal contour on the chest film in roughly 60% of patients with coarctation. The 'figure 3 sign' is the undulation in the distal aortic arch at the site of the coarctation (Figure 9-65). The distal convexity in this region represents the poststenotic dilatation. There is considerable variability in the size of the ascending aorta and in the upper half of the 'figure 3 sign.' The ascending aorta may be large,

Box 9-9 Anomalies Associated with Aortic Coarctation

COMMON

Bicuspid aortic valve with stenosis and regurgitation

Patent ductus arteriosus

Ventricular septal defects

Turner syndrome

RARE

Transposition of the great arteries

Double-outlet right ventricle

Shone syndrome (parachute mitral valve, supramitral ring, aortic valve stenosis, and aortic coarctation)

through the ductus will depend on the size of the ductus and the difference between the pulmonary and systemic vascular resistances. In this situation, the blood flow is frequently from the pulmonary artery to the descending aorta, a state that produces cyanosis in the lower half of the body. Oxygenated blood from the left ventricle goes to the aortic arch arteries, while deoxygenated blood from the right ventricle goes through the ductus to the lower body. A juxtaductal coarctation produces a complex pattern of blood flow, which may vary dynamically as the pulmonary and systemic vascular resistances change with daily activity.